MOM ON WHEELS

THE POWER OF PURPOSE FOR A PARENT WITH PARAPLEGIA

MARJORIE AUNOS, PHD

First Edition

ISBNs
eBook: 978-1-990688-05-8
Paperback: 978-1-990688-04-1

About the Publisher

Ingenium Books Publishing Inc. Toronto, Ontario, Canada M6P 1Z2.

All rights reserved.

ingeniumbooks.com

Edited by Marie Beswick Arthur, Boni Wagner-Stafford, and Amie McCracken

Cover Design by Jessica Bell Designs via Ingenium Books

PRAISE FOR MARJORIE AUNOS, PHD

As a wheelchair user for over forty years, I was not too worried to become a mother and trusted that I would be all right. That being said, there were many challenges, questions, unknowns, and let's be honest, many taboos. And very, very few tools and little help. Marjorie's book *Mom on Wheels: The Power of Purpose as a Parent With Paraplegia* is at the same time empowering and practical, and talks about parenting with a disability in a real and true voice. Being a parent is a wonderful adventure, and no one should deprive themselves of such an experience because of their disability.

—THE HONOURABLE CHANTAL PETITCLERC, PARALYMPIAN, SENATOR, AND MOTHER

I am humbled and honoured that Marjorie Aunos shared her profound inner transformation with me. She is a light to anyone seeking to build their resilience and well-being— even in the most difficult of circumstances. A must read!

—FATIMA DOMAN, SPEAKER, AUTHOR, COACH, CEO OF AUTHENTICSTRENGTHS.COM

Marjorie tells her tragic story in a tone that invites you in without bringing you down. In the end, she lifts you up. A powerful and critical exercise in perspective-taking. As a new dad, it moved me to tears.

—BRIAN MILLER, AUTHOR OF *THREE NEW PEOPLE*

Mom on Wheels is a story about one mother's struggle for dignity and support in a world that views disability as pathology and disabled parents as somehow incapable. It is a story about one mother's love for her son and her dedication to doing, as most parents do, what was best for him, even in the context of frequent barriers and experiences of discrimination. This is a story of one mom on wheels, certainly, but it is also the universal story of a mother's devotion and dedication.

—MICHAEL L. WEHMEYER, PHD, CHAIR, DEPARTMENT
OF SPECIAL EDUCATION, UNIVERSITY OF KANSAS

With steady, courageous guidance, Marjorie Aunos guides us into understandings of resilient and generative living that aid us not only in navigating the ups and downs of our particular lives, but in becoming better people: more thoughtful, compassionate, brave, and calm. She is both ordinary and heroic, imperfect and magnificent, and through her clear, heartfelt stories we are given the chance to become the same.

—MARIA SIROIS, PSYD, AUTHOR OF *A SHORT COURSE
IN HAPPINESS AFTER LOSS (AND OTHER DARK,
DIFFICULT TIMES)*

Don't be misled by the title of this book: it is much more than about a mom on wheels. This book is about a journey at life's crossroads filled with powerful love, outbursting self-determination, and a renewed sense of purpose. And it is also a tool you will want to pass on to the persons around you that you cherish the most.

—EVELINA PITUCH, OCCUPATIONAL THERAPIST, PHD CANDIDATE

After six years of running Speaker Slam, I can honestly say Marjorie is one of the absolute best storytellers we've ever had on our stage. I sat down to read a chapter, and finished the book in one evening. Riveting, vulnerable, honest, powerful, and INSPIRING!

I loved the honest, vulnerable, intimate journey into Marjorie's life-changing accident. Beautifully inspiring.

—RINA ROVINELLI, CO-FOUNDER SPEAKER SLAM

Mom on Wheels is so much more than a beautifully written memoir of adjustment to spinal cord injury; it is an exploration of what it takes to survive and flourish with a broken body in difficult circumstances. Marjorie gives readers an authentic account of the pain and grief that accompanies acquired disability and shows us what resilience, bravery, self-acceptance, forgiveness, and the support of family and friends can enable us to achieve. It's a book that reminds us that parenting is a shared challenge that doesn't need us to be perfect—just to love as we are able.

—SHANE CLIFTON, PROFESSOR OF THEOLOGY AND ETHICS, UNIVERSITY OF SYDNEY

Marjorie Aunos has openly shared her traumatic experience and its transformative effect on the course of her life without even a trace of self-pity. She tells her story with unusual perspective—this is not a blow-by-blow accounting of injury and living with a permanent disability. She gives the reader snapshots into the accident, her recovery, and adjustments in her life. She also expresses her fierce love for her son and how his presence in her life has motivated her over and over again as she's faced obstacles to living together successfully. As if all of this wasn't enough, she also seamlessly weaves in the devotion of her parents to support her and her son through their challenges. Her story alone is amazing, and her skillful storytelling makes this book a worthwhile read.

—C.A. GIBBS, AUTHOR OF *THE PICTURE WALL: ONE WOMAN'S STORY OF BEING (HIS) (HER) THEIR MOTHER*

We need this book now! The one guarantee I can make about this book is that if you read it, you will change some part of your life for the better. You might become a better parent, a better friend, a better caregiver, a better steward of our human family. But better and stronger.

—DR. RYAN M. NIEMIEC, SCIENTIST, PSYCHOLOGIST, BESTSELLING CO-AUTHOR OF *THE POWER OF CHARACTER STRENGTHS*

Marjorie draws you in with her compelling and authentic storytelling and then strikes you mentally and physically with the rawness of her experiences. I could not put it down.

This book is a loving homage to every strength of character that we know, and more. The passion and compassion is almost hypnotic. Don't start this book unless you have time to finish it in one sitting—or tremendous self-regulation.

This is a story of transformation. The unguarded telling of the author's story shows us that it is not just for ourselves that we do the things we do, but for the love of others—even when we do not know them.

—RUTH PEARCE, BURNOUT COACH AND SPEAKER, CIO
ALLE LLC

An essential addition to the literature as it invites the reader to look at the world through the elephant in the room: the cultural reality of ability-based judgments, norms, and conflicts. The message of this book applies far beyond the situation of the author. Everyone has ability expectations and is ability-judged by others, whereby these ability expectations come with personal and societal consequences. Then, with any unplanned drastic ability change (physical, mental, economically, social...) comes the need to question and re-invent ability expectations one has of oneself and others and others have of oneself.

—GREGOR WOLBRING, PHD, PROFESSOR, UNIVERSITY
OF CALGARY

This book is a cry from the heart—from a mother who has journeyed and survived catastrophic injuries—to all rehabilitation professionals, nurses, doctors, community workers, social workers, to everyday people everywhere, to law makers and government officials. It is a call for us all to see, to truly see, the everyday challenges of moms on wheels so that we can all become part of the solution (or simply get out of the way) and allow these committed and resilient mothers to get on with their job of mothering (without obstacles).

—CAROLINA BOTTARI, ASSOCIATE PROFESSOR,
FACULTY OF MEDICINE, UNIVERSITÉ DE MONTRÉAL

CONTENTS

I had a hard time falling asleep last night… I was thinking of that evening ten years ago: how I didn't know that my life was going to transform so drastically the next morning.

And then this morning, as I opened my eyes, I hallucinated. I saw a monarch butterfly clinging to the ceiling, for a few seconds, then flying off.

A butterfly is a sign of transformation, renewal, spirituality, and celebration. And a butterfly that flies off means change is embraced. A vision of a monarch comes from a guardian angel. A reminder that life is short and that we should forever be grateful.

I swear I didn't make this up! I guess this symbolizes the last ten years—and the next ones to come.

—Marjorie

THE CALL THAT NEVER CAME

I call her Star. Because in my eyes, that's what she was: A mama bear who would do anything to take care of her babies.

But her life circumstances tipped the odds against her. She had no other family to speak of and did not hold a job. She lived in a lower income neighbourhood—the only place she could afford.

The day I met Star, two child welfare workers were coming to her home to talk to her. She asked me to stay.

In that meeting, I saw a mom trying to follow what they were saying, fearful of every note they furiously wrote on their notepad in case it meant "bad mother, horrible mother."

Dirty laundry on the floor, *check*.

Broken toys lying around, *check*.

Her torture lasted more than forty-five minutes, during which three of us watched the way she bathed her son, how she tidied up her house (or didn't). She was being judged. And she frequently and desperately looked to me. For help.

Not once did the child welfare workers ask her *why* she did things the way she did, or *why* things were this way for her.

1

All Star knew was that they would take away her last child, her voice strangled by those notes on those pages.

Voiceless. Defeated. She had been reduced to a box they checked. Once there was a check mark, they stopped listening, because for them that box told a particular story: a story of neglect *in their opinion*, simply because Star had a disability, a diagnosis used against her as evidence to remove her children.

I worked with Star. And with so many others like her. I was there to assist, I was there to assess their progress, a psychologist supporting them and making sure they got the appropriate services. I always wanted to help out, doing as much as I thought I could, trying to ensure parents like Star would get a fair trial. Making sure they would keep their children in their own care.

Sometimes it worked. And other times, I felt helpless and powerless, only a witness to the gut-wrenching removal of their children.

So, when I became a disabled person, when my son was sixteen months old, I wept. I was terrified. I knew too well the stories of all those parents who had lost custody of their children *without any real evidence of neglect*. For no other reason than their disability.

It kept me up at night. At home, I would catch myself staring at the door, waiting for that knock, that call, for the questioning of everything I did as a parent. I would stare at the baby gate, wondering how the hell I was going to get it installed. I was incapable of leaving the house on my own, let alone of emptying out the garbage.

I would think of Star, whose disability and the lack of accessibility made it impossible for her to go down to the laundromat to wash clothes. Whose disability made it more difficult for her to pick up toys on the floor.

She was me. And I was her.

And I caught myself thinking: *Are those good enough reasons to remove a child? To remove… my child?*

But no one came.

No one.

Nobody ever knocked on my door. Nobody ever called my house. No one questioned my parenting. Nobody even looked.

I was a single mother with a recently acquired disability and I was scrambling to keep it together. Yet somehow society had determined, without any official assessment, without even meeting me, that my son was going to be safe in my care.

And even though it baffled me on the one hand, on the other hand I knew why.

I am a white, educated professional in the health sector—a psychologist, who teaches in universities and who holds a managerial position in a rehabilitation centre. I realize I'm privileged.

But I'm still just ordinary. I am an ordinary person who, a few months shy of her thirty-fifth birthday, a single parent of a sixteen-month-old, did *not* die from a life-shattering car accident.

But I did change. I sustained permanent loss of sensory and motor functions from below my armpits to my toes.

I became a paraplegic parent, no more and no less challenged by my parenting circumstances than Star.

But I couldn't scream about this injustice. *Not yet.* I still felt I needed to hide, just in case. They could still change their minds *about me.* So I was rendered voiceless—by the fear and the guilt that my son was still in my care.

And although the silence of the call that never came was deafening, it was also the beginning of something. A gentle explosion that made me aware that my privileged position and my disability status *together* would hand me the perfect megaphone to amplify the voices of others.

To show that disability alone does not impact our parenting.

But lack of accessible housing, lack of good paying jobs, and biased societal attitudes do.

I'm ready now. To be heard and to take a stand. To speak up, to ensure everyone is invited to the table and has a dedicated seat. Or at least a space of their own to park.

I want to make sure someone like Star never goes unheard again.

ONE
THE MAN OF MY DREAMS

I once loved a man more than words can say.

The Man was one of the sexiest—heck no, he was the sexiest man I had ever met. He was funny, sensitive, strong, kind, and generous. And he thought I was his sunshine.

Sometimes The Man and I worked on the same team of professionals, including social workers and me as the psychologist, assigned to assist families headed by a parent, mostly mothers, with intellectual and developmental disabilities (IDD). At the time, I was the only professional in Quebec with this particular expertise.

I loved my job. I was dedicated to being the best advocate I could be. I tried to think outside the box, to analyze and diagnose, to understand, to listen, and to support everyone involved, as much as I could.

The first case The Man and I worked on together was where a mom with IDD was fighting to retain custody of her son. The social worker assigned to the case was fighting an uphill battle and needed support. For this family, I was sworn in as an expert witness in her custody hearing. This is where I felt, for the first time, the power and influence of my standing, knowledge, and expertise. With my résumé, my research, my doctorate, and my publications, I realized I could change lives. My thesis had given me many ideas on how our society could better support families and orient services for the benefit of children and their parents. It was gratifying.

The Man and I continued to cross paths. We shared a common objective: to make things better for families. Our professional ethics, our unique abilities to fight for their right to self-determine and have a better quality of life had ignited a mutual understanding. And a mutual interest in the other.

If our interest sparked at work, we must have fallen in love on the dance floor. Dancing had been a passion since my ballet classes as a child. I always danced like nobody was watching. In dance, I let myself go. I was free… from stress and problems, but also free to be myself. Without hiding. When I was dancing, I felt confident and beautiful.

He was twenty-four years my senior and had children from a previous marriage. But it didn't matter. Our first official date was at Chao Praya, at the time one of the best Thai restaurants in Montreal. We shared a bottle of wine, our conversation flowing as it always did. Toward the end of our meal, I paused and told him how much I loved being with him. I loved talking to him. I told him that my one concern was that one day, I would want to be a mother. I would invest in a relationship only if he was open to having another child.

"I never thought I would have another child," he said, his response forever engraved on my brain. But my heart only heard the next part. "I also never thought I'd fall in love with a younger woman. When the time comes, and you want a child, we can talk about it."

And from there we went, on that road together. I was head over heels in love. I thought The Man felt the same about me. He certainly made me feel like the most beautiful woman that had ever walked the earth. I was my most vulnerable, sensitive, authentic self when I was with him. He was my destination, my end of the road. I had found the one I would be with for the rest of my life. He was mine and I was his. Period. No contest.

I loved my life. I was happy. For a head-strong, focussed, and determined woman who performed, succeeded, and achieved, it was exhilarating. Because for the first time in my life, I experienced passion in both my career and my personal life.

But as I approached my thirtieth birthday, I noticed a little hole in my heart. A tiny hole I had been able to ignore at first, but a hole that was getting bigger. It was starting to bother me. I was getting older and so was The Man. And I thought back to that conversation on our first date: I wanted to be a mom. So I asked him again.

And there we were, at an impasse. The answer to my question was a resounding "No." Which left me with a gut-wrenching choice: stay with The Man with whom I was deeply in love—or leave to pursue this intangible dream of motherhood.

I left. And my heart broke in the process.

TWO
GOING ROGUE

When I left The Man of my dreams, it was with the hope I would meet the love of my life. Leaving him was tougher than anything else I'd ever done.

My cousin Sylvia and her children were there, as they always were, giving me the love I needed.

Sylvia always had my back. She was my kindred spirit—the Prince Edward Island Diana Barry to my Anne Shirley. Her happy-go-lucky, deep, raucous laughter was contagious. With her magnificent curly ash-blond hair and zeal, she could energize a room—or get on everybody's nerves. She saw the good and the beauty in life. Sylvia told it like it was—especially if she disagreed. Clever, funny, and super strong—she was the definition of full of life.

Sylvia married young. She and her wonderful man, strong in his opinions yet kind and gentle, had two wonderful children. She once explained to me how much she loved her husband and how that love, although wonderful and powerful, was surpassed by her love for their children.

And then illness struck. Nobody understood Sylvia's symptoms. Doctors dismissed them as figments of her imagination or unimportant, until they couldn't—a morning when she woke half blind and couldn't move her legs. That week, she was diagnosed with metastasized breast cancer, the kind that does not forgive.

Three weeks before Christmas, doctors gave Sylvia six weeks to live. A force of nature, she pulled out the strongest weapon in her arsenal and, armed with immeasurable love for her two young children, she decided to beat the odds. Her goal: to live to the next milestone. One more month to her son's second birthday. Two more months until her godson's birth. Six more weeks until her daughter's sixth birthday. Each time, she asked doctors for more time to the next milestone.

Sylvia lived four years longer than the original prognosis.

Such is the power of love. And Sylvia. I turned to her in the darkest days after I left The Man.

Sylvia knew my heart had stopped beating and she reminded me it was still there. With her, I didn't have to hide my feelings, my thoughts, my despair, or my hope. She was my biggest cheerleader, reminding me to take steps forward, no matter how small. And so I did.

I dated other men. It was fun (no it wasn't) for a while. I always compared them to *him*. And I couldn't wrap my brain around the fact that I had left one man to become a mother, and now I was searching for another guy with whom I could become a parent. *"Hi, I'm Marjorie. I sort of like you. Do you want to have a child?"* I didn't think that starting a new relationship with the firm and sole purpose of procreating would end well.

My desire to be a mom was stronger than ever. While Sylvia continued fighting to stay alive, fighting for her children, I saw that I could also get back on my feet and find a way to enable my own dream of motherhood. If dating was not an option, I needed to find another solution. And I did.

I chose my sperm donor based on his essay, pedigree, personality, intellectual testing, and references. I chose him because he resembled most closely, on paper, a man I'd choose as a partner.

Trying to get pregnant via insemination was like riding a roller-coaster. There were the blood tests, the psychological preparedness tests, the PAP tests, one of which revealed some precancerous cells and surgery was required before I could begin the insemination. Through it all, I prepared my body. I did acupuncture to promote fertility. I stopped drinking coffee, ensured I ate well and according to nutrition experts. I tried to decrease my stress levels—although that part was almost impossible as I had taken on more responsibility and had started private practice. I endured moments of fear: what if I got sick, or I lost my job, or I didn't have enough money, or my baby got sick? I would be the sole provider yet also the sole caretaker. How would it work if I needed to take time off to care for him or me? Those thoughts brought doubt, but also brought me the resolve of knowing I could only do the best I could with what I've got.

The first, second, and third insemination attempts went... and failed. As I contemplated giving up on this crazy plan, Sylvia was undergoing brain surgery. She wasn't giving up! If she could keep going for her children, then I could keep going for mine.

Around attempt number seven I met with my doctor and shared the notes I'd been keeping about my fertility signs. I concluded I was being inseminated too late: I had a shorter cycle of twenty-six days versus twenty-eight so I needed the insemination procedure on day fifteen, not sixteen. The doctor didn't think it would make a difference, but I decided to go rogue and I listened to my gut.

On November 29, 2009, in a hotel room in Ottawa, after months of trials and tribulations, I found out I was pregnant.

Thomas arrived more than a week late, on August 12, 2010.

Sylvia died on October 25, 2010. She had just turned thirty-five.

Life after her death was gloomy. The family grieved and went about doing their best to support Sylvia's husband and children. She and I had dreamed of raising our children together and I had promised her that I would be there for them beyond her passing.

As we were figuring out how to celebrate Christmas that year, my baby—Thomas—was diagnosed with a ventricular septal defect, a hole in his heart. I felt guilty. I'd made him when I still had a hole in my heart that hadn't yet healed from leaving The Man, and I thought I'd transferred the hole to Thomas.

Thomas was six months old when he had open-heart surgery. Seeing him go through surgery so soon after Sylvia's death was difficult, but the care he received was phenomenal and he has recovered fully. The scar on his chest reminds us how fragile and precious life is. Every day I pull him close, turn my cheek to his chest, and drink in the wondrous soothing sound of his beating heart.

With his recovery, the future was once again looking up. My brother had gotten married, and I had moved on from The Man, no longer pining or hoping that the relationship with him would come back. I was starting to date again, and life was getting happier.

But more dramatic change loomed.

THREE
TODAY IS A GOOD DAY TO DIE
JANUARY 5, 2012

The sun was out, shining in a clear blue sky. We were coming out of a wicked snowstorm from the day before, and the light and warmth of the sun through the window felt rejuvenating on my skin. I was in such a good space. Just enjoying life and truly knowing how blessed I was. It was a little over a year that my cousin Sylvia had died and our hearts were healing: the pain wasn't as intense, although my thoughts of her were constant. My son was thriving and our family was strong. We had just spent three wonderful days together in my parents' cottage.

My parents' cottage is a wonderful place—two houses on a small lake in a tiny town ninety minutes outside Montreal with lots of space for both inside games and outside activities. My son was sixteen months old, and over these last few days we'd been sliding on a nearby trail with the older cousins and tubing on a small trail with the younger ones. We made a fire and cooked hotdogs. We wrestled in the fluffy snow, three grown women and several children trying to make my brother fall, without success.

We played video games; we ate marshmallows, laughed, and had so much fun.

I had decided that I'd go to work for a couple of days while Thomas stayed with my sister and my parents at the cottage. The festivities from the night before had run late and I was having trouble waking up. When I got up to the big cottage, Thomas was already eating breakfast in his highchair. His Cheerios were scattered on the tray in front of him like Lego pieces and his beaming face shot rays of sunshine into my heart. My brother and his family were also leaving that morning, so the house was bustling with people and preparations.

I packed and repacked my things, wracked by indecision over which boots to wear. I was headed into the city, where my nice, fashionable, leather, high-heeled boots made sense. But I was still in cottage country and those heels were not practical for the trek I still had to make between the house and my car. So I took them off, tucked them back into a suitcase, and instead pulled out and put on my big warm Canadian boots. I'd carefully chosen to wear my favourite purple sweater and jeans, the pashmina a friend had given me, and my black Columbia coat.

I said my goodbyes and walked up the hill. My mom followed and reminded me that I had said goodbye to everyone except to her. I hugged her, then pulled away saying I was already running late. It was not a proper goodbye.

I got into my car at 8:35 a.m., my luggage beside me and on the backseat. The route back to Montreal is not a complicated one: a small country road to Route 329, a road through the Laurentians that would take me to the highway. That narrow winding road did not intimidate me: I knew every twist and turn like the back of my hand as I had driven it a gazillion times. The road had already been cleared of the heavy snow from the night before and my car was adhering well to the asphalt. The drive felt safe.

I needed gas. I knew that at the corner of the country road and 329 heading south were two gas stations. I debated stopping for gas there, which would delay my already-late arrival at work. It was now 8:52 a.m., which would put my arrival at the office in Montreal at about 10:30, ninety minutes past my normal start time. While I knew very few people would be back at work that day, I'd chosen to go to work to get ahead on some files. That and the fact that I *sort of* had a date that evening—a nice home-cooked meal prepared by a really great guy—helped me decide not to stop for gas. After one last hesitation in front of the gas stations, I headed toward Montreal.

The fresh snow on the side of the road was twinkling like tiny little diamonds. Every so often, I'd pass another lake on the left-hand side. The forest was a constant on the right, sprinkled with the odd house. I was driving at the posted speed limit of eighty kilometres per hour on a road that looked and felt dry. A car behind me rode a little too close to my ass for comfort. I thought about how I could signal them to back off, but chose instead to focus on my own driving. Up ahead, a black pick-up truck was driving toward me.

Suddenly my car swayed to the left and my tires no longer hugged the road. My attempts to redirect my unresponsive car were useless. I thought of all the cars I'd seen on the side of this road over the last couple of months. *This is what's happening to me.*

As my car swayed to the right, I saw the black pick-up truck again, dangerously close, and remembered that car chasing my rear bumper. It was perfect timing. I realized a collision was inevitable.

I smiled—a little sarcastic one-corner-lift kind of smile one can have when fate is playing with them. Everything slowed down, except my thoughts.

FUCK. This cannot happen to my family again. Sylvia lost to us a bit more than a year ago and now... me? This is UNREAL. And unfair. My son.

My son is with my parents and my sister. They love him. My sister was at his birth and my parents spend a lot of time with him. He is happy around them. He will be okay. And my family… they are strong together. They know how to get through grief and loss. They will pull through together. But… me? Fucking crazy life.

I felt light and at peace. Death was coming for me and I was not scared. A bit pissed off that this was happening to me as I had so many plans for my life, but…

Today is a pretty good day to die.

I was as happy as I was ever going to be. At that moment, it felt perfect. I could return to my maker and embrace my cousin Sylvia. I knew she would welcome me with open arms. A vision of Sylvia's face swam before me, tears in her eyes. Why would she be sad to see me come?

Shit! It's because of my son!

If I died right then, Thomas would become an orphan. He already had no dad, and now, he was about to lose his mom.

I had not executed those conscious and challenging choices to turn him into an orphan, so I summoned all my energy and whooshed the Angel of Death away.

I am not dying today!

I was not dying because I couldn't. I'd made too many promises… to my son and to my cousin. I promised her, before she died, that I would be there for her two beautiful children, that I would love them as if they were my own, and that I would keep her memory alive for them.

Thomas. Marianne. And Maxime.

I said those names with all the love that there is in my heart. *Sylvia… help me pull through this. Make me survive.*

I closed my eyes.

Collision.

"Wake up!"

It was Sylvia, whispering in my ear.

I opened my eyes.

I had difficulty focussing. Not only had I lost my glasses during the crash, but my field of vision was narrow. I could see directly in front of me but everything was dark. I wasn't in pain, which surprised me. I was lying on my right side, held in place by my seat belt. It felt like my legs were extended, my feet touching the pedals.

Except I couldn't be sure what I felt. My legs also felt numb, as if they were swollen like marshmallows. It was weird, like nothing I'd ever felt before. Unnatural.

My legs… SHIT!

I felt tired as I tried to run a full diagnostic of my body and my predicament. I knew I needed to rest and conserve my energy as I figured out what to do next. Right then, there was nothing I could do.

I closed my eyes.

I heard a man's voice next. Opening my eyes slightly, I saw an undetermined figure out of the corner of my left eye.

Someone is here to help.

My eyesight seemed to be improving. In my peripheral vision I thought I could see another man walking toward my car. I could hear that he was trying to speak to me, but it sounded very far away and hollow.

My arms.

My left arm was by my side and my right arm was on the stick-shift. But I couldn't be sure because I couldn't move them. In fact, I couldn't feel them.

SHIT!

I could feel my heart, though, because it was sinking to my stomach. Pounding, pounding. Suddenly I started to freak out.

If I panic, it will make things worse.

I decided that my arms were more important than my legs—I knew I was not going to be running anytime soon.

But my arms… I need my arms. Focus.

SHIT.

I was scared. I really wanted my mom right then, but she wasn't there so I knew I needed to be a big girl.

I took a few deep breaths, and reminded myself I was loved.

Not being able to move my arms was *not* going to work for me.

I need my arms. I have my son to take care of.

I had asked to survive. I had cheated death for Thomas so I could raise him like I had planned. I needed my arms back.

With my arms, I know I will be fine.

And with this resolve in my heart, despite the little voice that was trying to tell me how serious this was, I turned to the only entity I thought might be able to help me out: I turned to God.

Please, give me back my arms. I will be okay if I have my arms. With my arms, I can embrace my son. PLEASE. GIVE ME BACK MY ARMS. I need my arms to take care of my son.

Tears streamed down my cheeks.

Oh… God… Please… Give me back my arms. I promise… I promise I will be okay if you give me back my arms…

And there it was. A little tingle in the fingers on my right hand. And then the same tingle on my left hand. I was moving my fingers.

It worked!

I tried to wiggle my fingers some more.

Stop moving! Are you crazy?!

I realized that moving might create more damage.

Don't move!

I kept my eyes closed, all my mental energy geared toward surviving with the least damage possible. I focussed on my breathing. Air going in through my nose. Air coming out of my nose. It was helping to calm me down.

Sylvia!

"Don't move," a man said. The man from the pick-up truck. "Help is on its way."

More time elapsed. First responders arrived. It sounded like many of them. I opened my eyes and recognized uniforms.

It took some time to get me out of that car as they wanted to secure my neck properly. They, too, believed my spine had been injured. When they finally got me out of the car, they put me on a gurney and into an ambulance. First to the nearest local hospital, where I gave my parents' phone number and doctors said they were sending me to a bigger hospital in Montreal.

How ironic.

Montreal had been my destination. I never thought I would get there with sirens blazing.

FOUR
WHO'S THAT LADY?

I t was five days after the accident before I asked my parents to bring Thomas to me at the hospital. Frankly, I didn't think I would be in the hospital for as long as five days—I was in deep denial.

I knew that Thomas would be frightened when he saw me in a strange bed with tubes octopussing all over... And he was. He clung to my mom as if his life depended on it. He refused to touch me, hug me, or sit beside me. He cried the full two minutes he was there, refusing to be comforted by me: his mom. I felt helpless and powerless that I couldn't be there for him.

It also hurt that Thomas kept turning to my mom—his grandma—for comfort. My mom was stuck in the middle. She needed to be there for Thomas and comfort him, but she also wanted to be there for me. I was her daughter!

And I felt angry—that my mom was going to get to take care of Thomas while I wasn't. I had wanted this child so badly and now I was forced to watch someone else raise him, or at least take care of him, in a way that I couldn't.

My mom understood all that. She knew that in order to get

through this, I needed to be his mom, even if I didn't know how. And so, she brought him to see me in hospital every day.

After the first few visits, where Thomas would cry for the whole visit, refusing to leave my mom's arms or sit on my bed, my mom had an idea. She started bringing his highchair! This seemed to work. Thomas and I did puzzles, played with blocks, coloured in his colouring book, and looked at picture books together.

My parents would stay close to us at first. Then they'd stay on the other side of the room, then outside my hospital room door. Close enough to intervene if needed, but far enough and out of sight so that Thomas could get reacquainted with me, his mother.

Sixteen-month-old Thomas loved to throw the toys my mom brought. He threw the toys, looked at them, and then looked at me. I'd look at the toys and then look at him. I did not pick the toys up—because I couldn't. All I could do was shrug.

My dad started to come in and pick up the toys. But that became a repeating game on its own. Mom and Dad and I agreed they should only intervene for safety reasons or if I called them. I needed to do things, to make decisions for him and I, and Thomas had to learn that things would be different with his mom from now on.

For the first five and a half months, my parents lived in my house with Thomas. They felt he would be less traumatized if at least he had the same bed and the same house and the same routine.

Everything was changing for him. For me. It felt important that he knew some things would remain the same. My love for him, for example. A child that young gets attached to the person who gives them daily care, the one who comforts, the one who rocks them to sleep, hugs them, kisses them. So we needed to find a way for me to be able to do all that, or at least to be part of the process.

After six months of rehab, I came home for the first time since the accident. I was overwhelmed: with joy at being back home with Thomas, and with fear over how I would manage in a home that wasn't adapted for a person in a wheelchair. I had no idea how I was going to make it.

It was a beautiful Friday at the end of May and we had people over for supper. The table outside was set and Thomas was playing in the yard, which was dotted with his playthings: a sandbox filled with tiny shovels and buckets, a tricycle, and a small plastic toy slide.

Thomas wanted to slide but, because my wheels couldn't navigate the toys and the grass, I asked my dad to stand behind Thomas in case he fell. As we hadn't really figured out what we needed to do together to coparent, my dad discarded my request, saying it wasn't necessary because Thomas could climb up on his own. I didn't want to argue and, more importantly, I didn't know how to relay that I was his mother, and that I would normally have stood behind the ladder myself, but this was something I could no longer do. In that moment I needed him to do it for me.

Of course, what I feared would happen, happened. Thomas slipped on the top step and fell backwards. And all I could do, was sit there. In my wheelchair, just a few metres away, literally paralyzed, as I watched my son slowwwwwly fall backwards.

As I yelled, "Fuck, Dad! I told you this would happen!" it triggered a strong response. Dad stood up as fast as light and jumped forward to hold Thomas up with one hand as my son landed awkwardly onto the grass.

When I had asked my dad to be a surrogate for me, I truly was asking my dad to have my back. I needed him to be there for me and my son just like his grandfather had been there for him.

To understand what I mean by that, we need to go back in time... to 1941 in Nazi-occupied Paris. My dad was five months old and was sent to Normandy to be raised by his grandparents. His grandparents were raising their ten-year-old daughter while mourning the loss of their adult sun—my dad's uncle—a casualty of war.

My dad needed their love and they all needed the hopes and joy of a little man. It was a good combination. My dad often shared his memories of his grandfather, his *petit père*, as he affectionately called him, with whom he shared a special bond.

One story in particular sprung to my mind in the yard that day. It was the time my dad's *petit père* found my dad sitting on the edge of one of those famous white chalk cliffs in Normandy, with his feet dangling off.

Just a little boy, unaware of the danger, enjoying the scenery of his playground. My dad had recounted how his *petit père* had approached him, slowly and carefully, to coax him away from the edge and save him from a fall.

When Thomas fell that day, my dad realized what a precious gift life was giving him. For the second time in his life, he was going to be part of this magical diad of grandson and *petit père*, except that this time around, he would be the one holding the role of *petit père*.

And I was now sitting on the edge of my own cliff, facing an ocean filled with new challenges. An adult daughter, still needing her dad to be there for her.

Being a parent is a lifelong commitment. We cherish our children, and our children's children. We protect them from harm, hoping that in the process we can teach them to stand on their own. But sometimes they fall, and all we can do is buffer their fall and help them get back up.

Like my dad did for my son that day. Like he and my mom did for me.

My dad realized he would need to be more than just Grandpa. He would be my arms and legs when necessary. He needed to be my proxy parent on demand—my demand.

The partnership between my mom and me was more evident and natural. We didn't need to plan or discuss it at length. She instinctively understood what I needed her to do, how to do it, and when to back down or back away. And she knew that while she could have stepped into a mother role for Thomas on her own, she respected the space I needed to take back my role as mother, with a few modifications.

One example was bath time. Safely giving Thomas a bath was impossible for me in the toddler years as I needed at least one hand to hold onto my wheelchair so I wouldn't fall. Mix a wiggly toddler with soapy water and you get a recipe for trouble. We team-parented through that routine with brilliant intentions.

The deal was that my mom would follow my directions while she was washing Thomas. During bath time, all three of us would be in the bathroom. I'd say something like: "Mamie, I think Thomas needs to have his hair washed today. Could you take some shampoo and wash his hair for me please?" I'd then turn toward Thomas. "And Thomas, don't forget to close your eyes as Mamie is putting some shampoo on your head!" When things were awkward, or when it didn't work because Thomas was uncooperative, for example, Mamie would alert me. I could then adjust my directives to fit the situation.

Along the way, sometimes my parents followed my directions. Sometimes they'd push back and say something could not be done the way I'd directed. And I needed to learn to trust their instincts and to remember that they'd raised children before, so they actually had more experience than I did. Yet we learned that my son was often more compliant when directives came from me, or they reflected the way I would do it. I knew what was best for him. And he trusted me.

We all had to learn to communicate with each other better, to treat each other with compassion, and to know that we were each trying our best.

We soon learned to be grateful for the fact that our feeling-off days didn't all come at the same time: when Dad was low energy and exhausted, Mom and I seemed able to pick up the slack; when I needed a break, Mom and Dad were there to fill the gaps, and so on. We were learning to be a team, supporting one another.

We also had to learn what our roles were. We needed to have clear boundaries—and when we crossed them, to apologize.

FIVE

DREAMING OF DANCING

Drums sound. Rhythm is in the air. People are laughing and singing, or maybe singing and then laughing, having fun.

The stage is filled with performers. The tables and chairs arranged in front are filled with guests. There is an open bar to the side. Active tenders juggle silver shakers and create unpronounceable elixirs, and pour straight liquor over icy rocks. The place is alive with possibility.

Back to the stage, where the band plays a popular song by Enrique Iglesias.

¡Bailando! Dancing!

My family is here—all of them, young and old. And a few dozen friends. They all have wide smiles. They laugh and point to the stage.

My brother, the extrovert (especially after a few rum and colas), is moving his hips and feet in cadence with the beat of the drums. He really wants to win that bottle of rum the organizers have promised:

"Take your turn on stage! Convince the crowd you are the best dancer and you'll win a bottle of fine Cuban rum!"

I don't know why this is so important, because this is an all-inclusive resort, but my brother is competitive and he wants to win.

But he hasn't won yet. Oh, no, because I... I... am the competition. And I want to win! And dancing is my cup of tea! I will convince the crowd that this honour is mine. I take my turn on stage. And I dance, and move, and twirl, wild and free.

¡Bailando!

A nd then... I'd wake up. Post-accident, my dreams were still filled with the old me—or who I should have been. Each new day a fresh and painful reminder there was a whole new reality.

Right before my accident, I had it all: my baby, my family, my friends, a job that allowed me to contribute and to make a difference in the lives of others. My life had meaning through my work, but also through my connection with those I loved and in how I experienced life.

After my accident, I was ashamed over what I saw as my inadequacies as a person with a spinal cord injury using a wheelchair. I felt I would be a disappointment (mostly to myself) if I didn't or couldn't do and perform like before. I didn't want to face the harsh reality: if I lost my ability to perform at work, on top of everything else I'd lost, what would this mean? Who would I be?

Our names have a long history of labelling our function in society. The blacksmiths, locksmiths, and gunsmiths bore the surname

Smith. The carpenters, bakers, and millers were identified by their life's work. Waggoner, painter, mason. The Middle Ages brought about a sense of identity that was wrapped in the honour of a profession, the pride of a skill. Our names indelibly connected us to who we were.

I *was* my work. My identity was wrapped up in my job—*I was a psychologist*. Going back to work had normalized a part of me and unraveled what I hadn't even begun to knit together. I hadn't wanted to see that I needed to actualize myself following change. I needed to find ways to embrace what changed, but all I could do was deny it.

I should have taken the time to reflect and plan my next moves, but I didn't. I couldn't. I couldn't face that dark pit that had formed below and in front of me.

And each night I dreamed I was dancing.

Were these dreams a sign I was actively avoiding the grieving process? Was my mind creating diversions to escape the inevitable? Was I surfing feelings when I needed to be feeling them? These were some of the issues raised in therapy sessions after the accident—but unlike my physical therapy sessions, these mental health sessions made me feel worse. So I resisted, denied, and avoided some more.

Like many who have suffered a traumatic accident that changed their lives, the answer for me was yes to all of the above.

Surfing my feelings might be a good strategy when I'm managing a panic attack, but surfing feelings to avoid ever having to face the facts behind the feelings is not.

My problem was this: I was denying their existence and, through that, I was denying the grief that was right there, all the time, waiting to be processed.

I never wanted to look at my feelings head on. If I did, it might produce a tsunami of fear that I was unprepared to deal with. Like asking me to eat a whole side of beef in one sitting. I couldn't digest everything at once. I never wanted to look at what the accident had done to me. *To me.*

At first, I saw myself as a victim of my accident. Someone who was powerless or helpless. If this had happened to me, it must have been because I deserved it. Because I wasn't a good enough person. Because I was a bad girl. It must have been my fault in some way, otherwise... *why?*

Maybe I was being punished. Maybe it was because I always felt so sure of myself. Maybe it was to teach me a lesson. Maybe if I had been a better person, this would not have happened.

All these thoughts compounded into feelings of self-loathing, sadness, bitterness, and anger.

My rehab team determined I needed psychological support services and assigned a psychologist to me. And I didn't like the service I got.

As a psychologist, my approach had always been from a cognitive behaviour perspective: a situation occurs to us, our thoughts then impact how we view or perceive that situation, and this affects the feelings and emotions attached to it.

A psychologist employing the cognitive behaviour approach may have helped me identify those thoughts, to work on them and challenge their validity.

The psychologist I saw at our rehab centre was not from the school of cognitive behaviour. She was new and less experienced than me. At least that's how I saw her, whether or not it was true. In our first session, I felt like she made me speak about the accident. The truth was that she asked me to speak about whatever I wanted. I thought the accident was what I needed to talk about, so for the whole hour, I spoke of every single loss I'd suffered as a result of the accident. I cried. I wanted to die. I thought that I should have asked to die, that day in the car, instead of asking to live. The renewed rush of pain and despair all that talking brought on led me on a downward spiral and closer to the abyss. *Why had I survived?* I was a burden on everyone. Just a dead weight.

The psychologist just listened. She didn't interject. She didn't challenge my thoughts. She didn't help me see my strengths. She didn't support me in a positive manner. She just sat there. All the good that an hour of physical therapy produced for me she undid. In one hour.

At least that was my perception. It was what I told myself.

I went back a second time but it was no better. My mood, my motivation, my reason to work out and get active were lost, like a leaf in a hurricane.

I never went back. I fired her. And the one after that.

Grief is like an old friend that comes to visit every now and again, bringing with it gifts of comfort and sorrow.

Intellectually, I knew that feeling grief was required to move on. Somewhere deep inside I knew that I needed to get to a place where I could accept that things were different—that I was different. But I would not let myself see that and I could not let myself feel it.

Even if I could magically walk again, my perspective had been changed forever. I tried to go back to the place before my accident. That old me didn't exist anymore and I needed to accept that.

But I refused.

I denied that my disability had to affect every area of my life—including work.

By avoiding the mourning process, my old self prevented me from ushering in and then getting to know my new self.

Grief is like a well-travelled, eccentric aunt who begs to be accepted for who she is. When she comes to visit, her ways are a necessary invasion in order to show us things she's brought from the far corners of the world, some of them quite disturbing but they are things that gift us wisdom.

Grief can lead us to reexamine our identity.

Who was I?

Who am I now?

Who will I be?

Why was I born?

What was my purpose?

What is my purpose?

What am I meant to do or be?

What makes me, me?

So many questions.

As I struggled to accept my new limitations, the new questions about who I was and who I was going to be seemed unanswerable. Insurmountable.

After the accident, not only did I feel cheated because I was not able-bodied anymore but, over time, I found it hard to feel part of a new crowd. I kept comparing myself to the best over-achievers of my newfound community. Chantal Petitclerc and Rick Hansen are two of the most honoured Canadian Paralympians. Petitclerc is a champion wheelchair racer, a world record holder, and holds a seat in the Canadian senate. Rick Hansen is best known as the Man in Motion for his twenty-six-month, 40,000 kilometre journey around the world in his wheelchair, but he's also founder of the Rick Hansen Foundation and advocates for a world without barriers for disabled people. They seemed to have it all figured out.

Both Rick and Chantal suffered spinal cord injuries, like me, in motor vehicle accidents. But they were both teenagers when they lost the use of their legs. While I knew it must have been hard to adjust at such a critical time of their development, I told myself that because they were so much younger, they somehow included being on wheels as part of their identity. I, on the other hand, had constructed my identity over thirty-four years—without wheels. I couldn't relate.

There were other examples of people with physical limitations from birth... people with a strong identity. There was no before-and-after story for them—there had always been and there would always be things they could do and things they couldn't. There was no change to adjust to.

Almost everyone I compared myself to became a parent. A parent with a physical disability. Just like me. How could they be happy as parents without even a murmur about their physical status? I felt inadequate because I was Not Happy being a parent with a physical disability. I felt angry. Sad. Mad. Furious.

But mostly, I was lost.

Nobody was like me. Nobody was a successful over-achiever who then lost it all because of a car accident. Nobody had to face the dreadful rehabilitation process while parenting at a crucial time of their toddler's development.

My concept of my mothering role had been crushed. And grieving that role led to a series of losses that it seemed would never end. Every struggle became a new loss.

With each loss I became less and less connected with others around me, others like me, others like the before me.

All I wanted to do was curl up in a ball. But I couldn't. I had a toddler to raise. I had to make tough decisions for our future—like where we were going to live and how, as our old house had stairs. On top of that was a full-time battle with insurance companies.

Each day I faced new limitations, new challenges, new losses.

Rehab was where I learned what I could still do, but it was also where I was reminded of all the things I couldn't do anymore. Anyone who said, "Look at the glass half full," received the same response from me: "Fuck you."

Becoming paraplegic was not only about losing the ability to move my legs, stand up, and walk. With paraplegia came a cascade of secondary losses. And I think those losses hurt the most, as they were unassuming until I saw their impact.

I will never accept the fact that I lost the ability to walk, to control my bowels and bladder, or the dramatic impact on my health. Accepting limitations has never been me. What I do accept is that I can manage with what I have while I work to relinquish my anger and sadness. I can also focus on what I can do to make myself more independent, while letting go of the things I cannot fix on my own.

As a person with a spinal cord injury, I needed determination to reach new ways of being independent. I needed courage to deal with ongoing pain that comes as physical and emotional hardship. And I needed patience, without which I'd have little self-control and barely any humility.

I had to stop comparing myself to or competing with others. I had to accept being myself, and to learn this was enough and just right. But for that to happen I needed to recognize my own vulnerabilities.

Everyone grieves and mourns differently, and at their own pace. For me, grieving the old me meant taking action. In my own time. It meant I had to find what was right for me. My grief is as unique as my eyes, my palm, my fingerprints. I'm the only person who really knows what I need.

And I needed to accept the fact and importance of the grieving process.

I learned to allow myself a full range of emotions by reminding myself that grief and joy can exist in the same space. I learned that sadness, feelings of loss, or anger could hijack any moment, that grief often comes at the most inconvenient times—aren't they all inconvenient?

Through therapy and reflection, I realized that it had become impossible for me to tackle all of the roles I had been holding on to (like work) and be healthy. The realization that I could no longer strive and excel the way I used to, at each of my roles, both petrified and destabilized me. My accident had created a new victim: me at my core, psychologically and emotionally.

To roll forward, I needed to be able to close some doors behind me in order to see the ones opening in front of me.

Nine years post-accident, I got to contemplate and reflect on who I wanted to be. The questions that had been paralyzing me with fear began to offer a glimmer of hope for the future. "What was I supposed to do now?" became a harbinger of an even deeper purpose, as I could be an even stronger advocate for disabled parents when I was one myself.

But first I had to crash and burn—emotionally.

SIX
SEVEN GLASSES

As I self-identified with work, trying to keep up the same level of quality services our team had always delivered, I worked more than I should have. I still wanted to be everything and do everything I thought I was supposed to, just like before. I had dived into my work to hide the fact that my accident had changed me. My stress level quintupled.

Going back to work so soon after my accident—about six months—came about because my mom was desperate to ease my desperation.

On the days I had no distractions, no physical therapy, and no visit from Thomas, anguish would drive me to hide my head under the covers—I would literally pull them up over my face. Finally, Mom suggested I go back to work.

I ran through the scenario in my head.

Being a psychologist and manager, I spent most of my time in a chair. *Check.*

I sat at a desk, in front of a computer. *Check.*

I used pens and paper. *Check.*

I generated ideas, and had the capacity to find solutions. *Check.*

So every Monday, my mom or dad would drive me to and from the office (driving was something I never wanted to do again, ever) where I spent four hours getting used to being back at work. Not fully back in my pre-accident role, but as a kind of intern.

Back in my old office. *Check.*

Back with my friends and colleagues. *Check.*

Feeling like I could contribute again. *Check.*

Doing everything to measure up to the old me. *Check.*

Four hours was the longest I could manage at the office as the toilet facilities were not yet adapted for me in my wheelchair. Soon that changed. But in the spring of 2013, another wrench was thrown in the works: my boss announced she was being promoted.

Scared that my new boss would not understand my needs. *Check.*

Scared I would not be supported in the continuing return to my job. *Check.*

Sad because I would not be working as closely with my boss, who was my friend and mentor. *Check.*

Devastated because I wouldn't be able to follow in her footsteps and apply for her job. *Check.*

Crushed because I wanted to have her old job. *Check.*

If I hadn't had the accident, it would have been the natural next step for me to apply for it. From my wheelchair, with my physical needs and limitations, I felt as if I couldn't.

I went to see her in her office to congratulate her. When she announced she would accept my candidacy, I cried. I told her it wasn't possible with my being in a chair.

"Why? What are the obstacles you see?" she asked.

For each obstacle I named, she found or suggested a number of solutions.

For. Every. One.

She was willing to make the adjustments necessary to ensure I could apply for and do the job.

Which was how I became the director of professional services.

In those first few years, my work was my lifesaver. I thought everything else would fall into place as long as I was working. The job centred me, permitting me to be creative in my contributions and to feel connected to others.

Each of my colleagues made some sort of sacrifice: some took on a little more work, others traded tasks with me. My disability hadn't affected my capacity to think, but it had affected my stamina. I simply couldn't work under pressure for long periods of time the way I could before my accident. But I tried to deny it and pushed through.

What I didn't realize was the impact the job would have on my overall health. I was blinded by my need to carry out my perceived purpose, to answer my calling.

First, I gained weight, which triggered a corresponding loss in my arm power and cardio capacity, in my physical mobility, balance, and posture. Pain developed and lingered in my shoulders and neck. More importantly, the physical energy deficit affected my time with Thomas.

For more than two years I prioritized my work, forgetting to take care of my physical and mental health. The weight gain continued to prevent me from being autonomous. The shoulder pain prevented me from taking part in certain activities.

No hobbies. *Check.*

No activities that triggered positive emotions. *Check.*

Undatable. *Check.* (Why would anyone be interested in me like this?)

Lonely. *Check.* (I lost friends who couldn't handle my new reality.)

Late getting home. *Check.* (Often, my adapted transport was delayed.)

A bad mom. *Check.* (Focussed on and stressed out about work.)

All I wanted to do was go to bed or work some more to catch up. So, I'd yell at Thomas and rush his evening routine. I couldn't wait for him to sleep so I could return to my computer or answer a call.

At work, I regularly had to change clothes and diapers due to incontinence. Nobody knew that the couch in my office was not really meant for them to sit on during meetings; it was a place for me to change my clothes when I needed. Being late to change the catheter meant a higher risk for UTI and incontinence, which would stop me from doing activities outside of the home for up to a week. If wet for a long time, I was at higher risk of developing a pressure sore, which could mean having to stay in bed for months until it healed properly.

I didn't fully appreciate the mental energy it took for me to manage my health, what and how much I ate, the number of transfers (from wheelchair to car, for example) I could do per day, how much water I drank, in addition to the mental energy of being a single parent and a senior manager. I didn't prioritize self-care for myself and everything became too much for me to handle.

And then a bomb hit: the whole health and social services system was about to change, people important to me disappearing into early retirement, or taken to other jobs. My boss no longer my boss. Nobody who knew who I was and what I could contribute. Financial cuts leading to service cuts were coming, and I understood the impact on clients, families, and staff. I saw myself as the last pillar left holding up a building. I was again confronted with the limits my new condition had brought.

Sitting in my office, door closed, alone, in the dark, bawling my eyes out, I realized that for months I had been saying goodbye to members of my team who were leaving, while receiving a pile of their dossiers. Staff who were staying would knock on my door and cry about all the changes we agreed did not make sense and were bad for clients. For months, in between these knocks, I would close the door, turn off the light, and cry, unable to stop. Until the next knock or the ping on my phone reminded me of the next meeting.

I had never really stopped working, and I'd continued to say yes to every opportunity, regardless of my new physical and psychological conditions. I never took time to recharge, to observe what my injury could mean, and it was backfiring.

Then I fell off my high horse. I had burned out. I was having a mental crash leading to adjustment disorder, major depression, delayed post-traumatic response, and generalized anxiety. I went on leave.

Although burning out is not the best way to go, it was a blessing in disguise because it led me to readjust my priorities.

By holding on to the before-accident me, I failed to prioritize self-care. I stopped moving my body, incorrectly thinking that movement wasn't important for my paralyzed body. But not moving makes a body stiff. Every body. Not exercising eroded my strength and chipped away at my stamina. As my body got stiffer, my mind got weaker. Not being active affected me mentally more than I could have imagined—my mind wouldn't work and my words were coming out all jumbled. But I still needed to feel productive.

So I reintroduced a workout routine in my life. I started slowly, a few minutes per day on my hand bike. I increased the duration until I was able to hand bike six times a week for one hour. I added exercise once per week on the GEO, a walking machine that resembled a treadmill but with a harness, holding me in a standing position while the treadmill forced my legs to move as though they were walking. This gave me a chance to stand up and sweat.

All this exercise increased my heart rate. But more importantly, the exercise gave me a purpose: to get my body healthy and my mind strong. When I worked out, no other thoughts crossed my mind. It provided me with a sense of relief and release. It allowed me to be focussed and purposeful. It still does.

Rolling Forward with Self-Care

Energy is like water in a glass: if I spill too much one day, I won't have enough left for tomorrow.

Every week, in the bank of me, in my account of my strength, I carry a gallon of water that represents the amount of energy I have for each of the seven days ahead. I have an empty glass for each day of the week.

I have learned to choose which of the seven glasses I fill with water (energy), knowing that if I pour all the water into the first three glasses, they will overflow and waste some of that precious water. And worse, there will not be any water left for the other four days.

So I choose carefully the amount of energy I spend (or save) for each day. If Thomas has an event or a show after school, I can choose to pour more energy into the glass for that day, as long as I plan for the next day to pour less.

When I don't prioritize my own needs, exhaustion kicks in and I become less patient, less positive, and more inconsistent. To stay available to my son, I have learned I need to stay available to myself.

The energy represented by the water analogy is more than physical. It's mental and emotional too. There's the energy to get myself ready each morning, and I also have to make sure Thomas is prepared. I have my own schedule and to-do list, and I have his too, juggling many schedule-balls in the air and ensuring everything is done, done well, checked off the list, and filed away. The load I carry includes being the financial and emotional provider, balancing my responsibility to work and earn a living, while saving and finding quality time to spend with my kid.

There is always a push and pull going on. What should I do first? Did I forget to do something? Where are my keys? Does Thomas have enough money on his lunch card? Should we go apple picking or does he have too much homework? During that mind-landslide I can be distracted enough that I break a jar of tomato sauce on the floor—and all that worrying gets slopped on the floor in a red goopy mess. My new priority is to clean my floor and avoid broken glass, as this could puncture my tires (for real).

If I'm not on top of my game, it is impossible to do or keep track of it all. When I am on top of my game, I can manage. And being on top of my game means I take time for me. Interesting dichotomy but, nonetheless, true.

I'm now better at remembering to plan for which days I will need to pour extra water into the energy glass and which I can pour less into. I have learned that I must take care of my own glasses of water first before I can be of value to others, especially to my son Thomas.

SEVEN
ONCE UPON A SECOND TIME

A few days after my accident, still hooked to tubes, the nurses and doctors caring for me wanted me to sit in a chair so that I could prepare my body and mind to stand, get up, or in some way be active. I wasn't yet in recovery mode, so getting out of bed was an ordeal.

First, I needed to be put in a body cast to hold my neck and spine in place to prevent further injury and to ensure the bone grafts would take and solidify. It took two people to do that.

While still in bed, lying down, I was turned on my side and held in place by one person. This allowed my back to be lifted from the mattress so that the second person could place the back side of the brace. Once placed, I was rolled over onto that brace. If adjustments needed to be made in regard to the posture I was in, I would be rolled on my side again, until the back brace was properly placed. Then they would place the front part of the brace and tie it with Velcro to the back end of the brace. Adjustments followed to ensure it would hold my neck and chin up.

Putting on the brace took at least ten minutes, as they also had to ensure there were no creases in my clothes that would create a sore.

Once the brace was settled, I needed to be rolled over on my side again so they could place a sling under my pelvis. The sling would allow me to be carried over to a nearby wheelchair. They would then prop me up with multiple pillows, holding my arms in place.

It was not only the most uncomfortable position I'd ever been in, but to me it resembled torture devices from the Middle Ages. I explain it as dismemberment, which I know means being cut up, disassembled, pulled apart. The pain was more intense than when I had delivered my son—which had been excruciating.

The biggest issue was that once placed in the wheelchair, the staff would be busy with other patients. And I could not move on my own. I was in a brace that restricted my head, preventing it from moving independently from the rest of my body, while the rest of my body was paralyzed. Within five minutes I was moaning.

Moving one inch might cause the pillows propping up my arms to fall, which would cause way more pain as I didn't yet have the strength to hold my arms on my own. When I was kept more than twenty minutes in the chair, my moaning would shift to shouts: I would ask anyone passing through to help me.

Despite calling out and using the bell, I would often be left in that position for two hours—the time it took for rounds. When I refused to go in the chair, staff made it clear that if I didn't go in the chair it would delay going to rehab, as rehab was only for people who could sit in their wheelchair.

In any case, the first time I was positioned to sit up was in ICU. I was kept in the chair for about one hour, but since I had my nurse present, she kept changing and adjusting my position to prevent pain. To pass the time, I had asked her for some paper, a pen, and a clipboard. I needed to write what was in my head.

Three days post-accident there were a few thought-reels stuck on replay: reliving the car accident, thinking about the future—so many thoughts that I was compelled to get out onto paper.

From that chair, the first thing I wrote was a letter to the son of the ICU doctor who was treating me. The doctor knew our children were of similar age. My circumstances had touched him. He was doing long hours in the ICU, staying seven days away from his son every time he was on shift. I wanted his son to know how wonderful his dad was in treating his patients and what that did for "us"—those who received care from him. Writing that day helped me focus on something other than excruciating pain. Writing liberated me, helped me heal, and continues to do so.

For years I wrote every day, some days more than others. I'd write when events or struggles occurred, when surprised by happy moments; I kept journaling my life—my journey through spinal cord injury recovery. Six years later, I compiled those entries into the first version of this book. A year later, I revised the content and format of the book substantially, as I further processed new insights and adjusted to the events I'd previously described. Then I revised it a third time—before I found a publisher.

Each major revision led to new understandings, delivering more awareness: a new lesson here, a new lesson there. Each allowed me to literally renarrate my life, as I reworked each chapter.

And with each writing experience, I began to feel more confidence in the person I had become because of those struggles.

That is how writing became a healing tool.

As I got closer to the tenth anniversary of my accident, I felt this push to share my story, openly and with authenticity. As I shared, I became more aware of how my life had stabilized.

By that anniversary, I had come to realize that I physically needed help to raise Thomas in the early years, but that I hadn't needed help forever; it was situational—there was a timeline with a steady decrease of the physical help I required. By reviewing my writing I came to see that, even in the tough years, there were many joyful times. By having put my thoughts on paper, and later reading them, my strengths, bravery, and resilience were showcased, as was my post-traumatic growth.

In my new narrative I could choose to focus on my character strengths: the stuff that had helped me survive and recover. The strengths that had been developed *because* of my disability. I could ask myself: which elements of me had made me survive?

Through this, I was able to find and even recognize the different parts of myself. I didn't have to redefine who I was; I was already there.

The honesty of the pen—or the electronic pen (keyboard)— helped me deal with the feelings I had of being an imposter. I used writing to name that imposter—of the famous imposter syndrome —and once it had a name, I was better equipped to recognize that the strong and capable me was larger and stronger than the imposter.

Being honest meant stating I was nervous, scared, and sad, and owning that I was empowered, compassionate, and proactive.

Writing made me pay attention; it even helped me listen to others because, through writing, I learned to listen to myself. I fell in love with story. When we share our stories we understand ourselves better and leave a legacy for others, just as we are within overlapping legacies of others right now.

The type of narration we use gives us power over our emotions. Through a variety of ways to express ourselves, we essentially construct a story that impacts how we feel and, through that, we learn because our journaling, speeches, letters teach us.

It is not about discarding the tough times. It *is* about creating them authentically and placing them where they can reflect the light. And recognizing that for every tough time and negative emotion and challenging experience, there is an opposite or different view available if only we have the courage to turn around and look.

We can look at the rain clouds in the sky and think, *I hate the rain*. Or we can look at the rain clouds in the sky and think, *Rain is needed to make things grow. It's not always fun to get wet in the rain, but it is what allows the rainbow to pierce through the clouds.*

Rolling Forward Into a New Story

Participating in renarration brought me to a place of power, because I was now in control of what I would pay attention to within my story. I recognized that I could choose whether to focus on how terribly difficult it was to adapt after my accident or my cousin's death, or even my separation. Or I could choose to pay attention to the fact that I had adapted, that I had wonderful memories of people I had loved deeply, and that these experiences showed me that I could and should celebrate life and the fact that I have the chance to live it.

EIGHT
LET'S TALK ABLEISM

Being able means having control over my life and the choices I make. It doesn't have anything to do with being able to walk or stand. I *am* able and creative in finding new ways to live as a wheelchair user.

Every day I'm reminded that this world has not been constructed with people with disabilities in mind. Much of the world still says "the disabled," leaving out the people-first attribute. We live in a society that is predominantly ableist.

What does that mean?

At its core is the belief that people with disabilities require fixing. It defines folks by their disability. Just as racism and sexism harmfully classify, ableism promotes harmful stereotypes and makes inappropriate generalizations. Ableism describes those who operate from a foundation that regular, typical abilities are the best.

At organizational levels, ableism ranges from noncompliance with disability laws to segregation of students. It's lack of thought in inclusive building plans, and in many ways we haven't come far from the eugenics movement of the early 1900s, where scores of people underwent forced sterilization.

In today's everyday life, ableism is choosing an inaccessible venue for a meeting, running news stories that frame a person's disability as only inspirational, and the disrespectful act of using someone's mobility device as a hand or footrest. (Yes, people do that.) It even includes using an accessible bathroom stall when there's a nonaccessible one available—and how many of us have done that? A common ableist practice is to speak to an adult who has a visible physical disability as if they were a child, or even to decide to push a person in a wheelchair without asking or without waiting for them to answer when you ask if they need help.

Ableism involves all forms of expression that communicate a negative slight against people in an attempt to joke: "That's so lame," "You are so retarded," "Are you off your meds?" And comments such as "I don't even think of you as disabled, you seem perfectly normal to me."

That is the short ableism fact sheet.

To combat ableism, the single most important thing to do is make sure people with disabilities are involved in decision-making processes. But that's another book for another day.

But I needed to address ableism here because it plays an important supporting role in many of the concepts I was familiar with before my accident and then slammed up against afterward.

 Ableism is a set of beliefs, processes and practices that produce, based on abilities one exhibits or values, a particular understanding of oneself, one's body and one's relationship with others of humanity, other species and the environment, and includes how one is judged by others.

WOLBRING, 2008

I fell victim to my own internal ableist discourse. Values such as productivity, efficiency, rapidity, performance, perfection, and excellence were at the core of who I had constructed myself to be.

Ableism had become a central and crucial construct in how I defined myself. My core values based on ableism were associated with the concepts of overtime and overachievement and accomplishments in all spheres. Work had all my energy. Just like I gave myself fully to all aspects of my life: motherhood, homemaking, friendship, and family. Everyone got 100 percent. I was doing it all and I was pretty successful and proud of it, perhaps arrogantly so.

With the concept of ableism came the concept of beautyism. Although I never fit the criteria of the Victoria's Secret model, I always felt pretty. And I took care of my health and how I was presenting my body to the world. Ableism was ingrained in me and my understanding of where I fit in the world.

The results were devastating. Others were used to Marjorie-the-over-doer. I was used to Marjorie-the-over-doer. So, I faked it. I was an impostor and a fraud. I pretended every day that everything was normal. I went to work, I smiled, I laughed, I seemed happy.

But I felt dead inside, empty, ugly. It was a lonely place. A place and state that reinforced my fear of being unlovable.

Even my burnout was a front as I unconsciously hid the fact I had major depression and chronic PTSD with features of generalized anxiety.

And one day, it was time for me to see, really see, my true reflection in the mirror.

NINE
SHOULDA WOULDA COULDA

As an able-bodied person, I felt I could always say I was working toward perfection. And even when I fell short, I believed I still had a shot at it with all my experience and capabilities. I knew being productive and engaged in multiple projects made me visible to others. And being visible fed me a strange diet of external validation—because I valued the voices and opinions of others more than I valued my own. The approval of others confirmed who I felt I was. My successes showed me I was someone special and I thought I needed to be special to be loved.

Striving toward perfection meant I was always only as good as the last thing I had done; always aiming to add to my already long list of achievements, extending my numerous titles and roles, saying yes to all opportunities, becoming essential, irreplaceable. It's how I fed my self-esteem.

It was Autumn. All the golden leaves made their way from branches to ground. The night before had been Halloween. I'd had so much fun walking Thomas around the neighbourhood, teaching him how to be polite while trick-or-treating for candy. There I was, warmed inside and outside, layers of joy wrapped around me.

Of course, my dream life always predated January 5, 2012.

Upon waking from that dream, I thought: *if every wrong in the world had been righted, if everything in my world was right, I'd have been trick-or-treating side-by-side with my cousin, our children, and our moms. The men would have been home drinking beer, eating pizza, and handing out candies.*

The reality was: I had to wiggle myself and my wheelchair through a sea of people, then watch my son from a distance on the sidewalk as he rang each doorbell or called out "Halloween apples!" It was most distinctly not perfect.

The strategies that had served me well before the accident were rendered ineffective. Heck, they were making it worse. I over-thought everything: as a psychologist, I *should have* been able to prevent my own depression, anxiety, and post-trauma, or at least, I *should have* been able to reframe and rehabilitate myself already. A clinical psychologist, I *should have* gone into post-traumatic *growth*, not post-traumatic *disorder*. Every reflection led me to intense feelings of shame and disappointment. The *should haves* fuelled negative emotions which, in turn, increased my suffering.

My perceptions of perfection collided with the body I found myself in, which meant I could no longer uphold these standards. And that meant I had failed. Worse than that, it meant I *was* a failure. It meant I was no longer anybody. And it was all my fault.

The more I fell into depression, the worse I felt because it perfectly illustrated what I felt I had become: a loser. I over-focussed on my disability and what I could no longer do.

Six months after my accident I went on my first trip. For the first time since I'd been working in the field of parenting and parents with IDD, the International Association on the Scientific Study of Intellectual and Developmental Disability was being held in Halifax, Nova Scotia. I had been an active member of the Special Interest Research Group (SIRG) for fifteen years; I'd planned to attend from the moment the conference was announced years before.

At first I thought I couldn't attend. It was one of the first secondary losses that I cried about: I was going to miss out on the conference I'd been planning for so long to attend. I would miss out on seeing my friends and colleagues.

"We're going," said my mom. On a long list of things she couldn't fix for me, this was something she could easily fix for me. She knew that, with her help, I could find a way to go. I tried to resist, telling her all the reasons why it would not work, testing her theory of we-will-figure-it-out.

She came to my occupational therapy sessions and asked my therapist (OT) what we needed to do. We established a plan. The OT kept reminding us that things would surely happen, and the trip would be hard, but if we went with a positive, constructive mindset, we could make it work.

My dad found a hotel room with an adapted bathroom. We asked the airline how they could fly me there. We even rented a house in New Brunswick where we would vacation as a family after the conference.

The first week of July we flew to Halifax, and I attended the conference. To make sure I could get enough sleep, my parents offered to take Thomas in their room. After all, two able-bodied people would be more efficient at the bedtime routine than one person with a disability. Right?

As I was lying in bed, ready to go to sleep, all I could hear through the common wall was Thomas laughing and the squeak-squeak-squeak of him jumping on beds while Mamie and Pappy were telling him to "Come here!" and "No, Thomas!" as they tried desperately to get Thomas to settle down.

My mom and I were texting back and forth, me asking how it was going with Thomas, my mom admitting that they were having trouble. They had to pretend they were also going to sleep at 7:15 p.m. all in the hopes the two-year-old terror would finally doze off. She was texting me from under the covers.

I have since realized I'd have had better luck than my parents did putting Thomas to bed. My concept of perfect parenting got a significant reframe that day. It was a significant lesson that began to invalidate thinking that told me two able-bodied people could do a better job than a mom with a disability at imposing an evening routine on her two-year-old, even in a hotel room. I learned that day that even able-bodied people struggle in their parenting tasks. I saw how disability had nothing to do with the difficulties I was experiencing as a mom. Thomas was two years old and he was testing our limits. It had nothing to do with my wheels and everything to do with his developmental stage.

Every parent becomes battle weary, doubts themselves, and gets really, really tired. I was not alone. And my struggles as a mom had nothing to do with the fact I was in a wheelchair.

When I burned out (major depression, delayed PTSD, anxiety), I had been trying to be as perfect as before, parenting and working full time and teaching without properly adjusting to my new paraplegic reality. I told myself I needed to stay on course. And the only way to do that was to avoid the feelings and focus on the physicality. To get and stay physically strong enough and autonomous enough to care for him: my baby boy. I could deal with the feelings on my own time. I was a psychologist, and surely I would see the signs of despair and psychological illness when and if they crept in.

It was counter productive. It was destructive. Of course it backfired.

Letting go of all the things that were not helpful anymore was the biggest challenge of my life. But did it mean I needed to let go of my job? Of motherhood? I didn't want to find out in case it was that drastic.

I would have loved to be there for my son, physically in person, from when he was sixteen months to twenty-one months. That would have been perfect.

But I could not.

In truth, I was with him and he was with me every single minute of every single day. Because all my energy was geared toward our future together. All the work in rehab was channeled through my love for him. It was a fact: I couldn't be there physically with him until I relearned tasks that would make me autonomous in my daily living. Working hard in rehab gave my physical separation from Thomas a purpose. That purpose was to be as strong and independent as possible so I could parent him the best I could in our future. Not perfect, maybe, but perfect enough.

It was necessary for real growth to let go of the perfect parenting I thought I had to measure up to, to let go of the overachieving role I had filled in my career, the guilt for not giving Thomas the perfect life I had envisioned and promised us both. And it was essential I accept there was no crystal ball.

Who knows how I would have handled the terrible twos and threes or even the fucking fours and fives as an able-bodied parent? I would have struggled no matter what.

I had to dispel the idealized, alternate version of my able-bodied life. It was pure fantasy for me to believe being able-bodied made everything perfect and came with a guarantee of no struggles or issues to tackle. But, like many who have experienced a traumatic accident that leaves them in a perceived less-than-before state, I fantasized—and then some.

Then there was the guilt, anger, sadness, and despair. That had to go, too.

I had a perfectionist way of conceptualizing the world around me, inserting my perfect Before Self into it. I was an internalized ableist—judging and offending myself. To thrive, I needed to find the true authentic Marj and embrace how different she was from the Ableist Marj.

Rolling Forward Imperfectly Perfect

We are all doing the best we can.

This became my mantra. It helped remove some of the pressure. A lot of it, actually. The knot in my stomach that sometimes made me stop breathing, left. Gone.

This was my epiphany: we all struggle, we all face our challenges, and we all try our best. I knew this was true for others—I just needed to see it in myself. I needed self-compassion. And kindness. I needed to be kind to myself. If I could see my friends as being in the same storm as me, even if we were not in the same boat (or chair), I could see we were all rowing.

In my wheelchair, and from my wheelchair, I could still strive to be the best version of me, without engaging the perfectionist tendencies that were a self-destructive habit that most certainly led to my depression.

My journey would have to include working to accept the notion that the imperfect was, in fact, perfect.

It may be fear that demands we hold on, but it is wisdom tapping on our shoulder and asking us to let go.

TEN
PAINFUL PRIVILEGE

From the first moment I woke after the car accident, pain became a reliable, constant part of my life. I live with chronic pain of different kinds. These pains are different in sensation and intensity, are on all parts of my body, and are triggered by various things.

There are the pins and needles I can feel all over my legs, in particular on the soles of my feet, without being able to do anything about it. It is like a pricking pain, little dots of agony that come and go like heavy raindrops thundering on the inside of my skin.

A similar pain is located at the level of my injury, dorsal vertebrae T2, as if I had a centimetres-wide elastic band right under my armpits that runs all the way around my torso. It forms a constant discomfort, an irritation that won't ever go away. It is on that elastic band that sudden, sharp surges of intense, excruciating, raw pain arrive as if someone is repeatedly stabbing me.

Other times, it can feel as if blisters are forming—like my skin had been exposed to an open flame. Any soft touch—any movement, really—makes the pain worse.

Then there are my head, neck, and shoulders. Independent parts of the body that come together to host a headache of severe intensity. From time to time, after a heavy workout or due to improper positioning in my chair or incredible stress, I get horrific tension headaches. Those headaches start with severe throbbing stemming from my neck that climbs right up to behind my eyes. This pain is completely debilitating. I can't think. It makes it hard to breathe. I can't even keep my eyes open. All I can do is hold my head, curl up into a ball in my bed, and rock like a baby as I try to make it go away. In those times, I can't take care of myself or my child. All I want is my mom, to be held and rocked by her.

The torturous headache pain can last for hours in the intense phase, then for days it recedes to the background where it tells me it is getting ready for a second round. My neck and shoulders also have their own particular pain—their own private club, so to speak.

Of the plethora of pressure points in my shoulder area, some are right next to my scar, alongside my spine, where the screws were inserted during my operation. Then there is the pain in the middle of the shoulder blades, and points right under the armpits, where my back muscles attach. There are also the tiny pectorals, in front of the shoulders that attach the breast muscles to beneath my armpits. All of those small muscles that are so useful and necessary for most of my arm movements cramp or tighten up from time to time. Release of tension in those areas is sometimes achieved with an elbow massage or a hard massage ball.

Without having studied the muscle and nerve system of the body, I can tell exactly the path of the three nerves that give sensation and feeling to the arms. I have mapped the pain too many times to count.

Along with irritated hands, I can feel a pinch come from my neck, through to the elbow and planting itself in the hollow of the hand. Those same hands that cramp and numb. When I overuse my thumb, due to push-ups I regularly do from my wheelchair, or intense rolling, the hand and thumb pain is excruciating—feels like a bruised thumb, especially where the "cushion" of the thumb is. This is where the carpal tunnel is—I know this because I learned its location when I couldn't put any more pressure or weight on it.

And next: there is also the path from the exterior of the shoulder to the corner of my elbow to my wrist. This path is often sore, significantly more painful when my tendinitis leads to muscle weakness.

All of these sensations have the power to take my breath away. They bring me to a place where I can no longer think about anything except to try to prevent myself from screaming.

Then there are the phantom pains I get in my legs (around the joints mostly) or in my abdomen. The pain in my leg is an intense growing pain as if my leg is being taken apart… yes, as in dissected and bisected. The leg phantom pain shows up and stays for a few days at a time, preventing sleep. As for the ghost in my abdomen, well, she hung around a whole year. Despite all the poking and prodding and imaging, doctors could never find the source.

How many times can pain be mentioned?

I know you know the answer: an infinite number.

Pain is an interesting phenomenon because, while it hurts, obviously, and is viewed as something negative that we do not want to experience, I have learned that pain is like an alarm system. It's there to let us know when something has gone wrong or is about to go a kind of worse wrong. In that way, pain is a good thing.

I feel pain every single day. I feel different kinds of pain, at different moments, for varying lengths of time. Pain is now part of a chronic condition I have to live with. My pain is there to remind me something went wrong in that car, that I am paraplegic. (As if I need reminding!) So I need to live with it. And accept it for what it is. That's just how it is.

Years after my injury, as I was waiting for a meeting to begin, some of the clinical professionals in the room told me about a research project they were working on. It was related to the use of virtual reality. They offered me a try.

I put on some funky goggles that placed me in a virtual reality world. Visually, I had access to a world behind, to the side, and in front. I was then asked to look down at my feet and, as I did, I saw some legs and feet.

Then those legs started moving. My instructions were to imagine my brain was activating my leg muscles and prompting them to walk. Basically, I was concentrating on what it would feel like to be walking, and I was sending the signals necessary to walk. As I walked, the virtual reality program also provided sounds as if I had been walking. I was surprised after only five minutes of concentration—and *seeing* my legs move—many pain sensations had disappeared. When I finished the *walk*, the pain did not return and I was pain free for several days.

Rolling Forward through Acute Pain

But virtual reality research aside, pain is a reality I have learned live with.

I have learned that we suffer when we resist what is happening.

We don't want the pain. We don't like the pain. And so we resist. And what we resist persists!

Any type of pain will feel worse when I am stressed—and that includes the stress of being mired in thoughts of wanting things to be the way they were before.

We can find ways to deal with all discomfort—from agonizing physical pain to emotional distress—by being curious. When I approach it with curiosity and lean into the pain or discomfort, there can be a shift. Releasing the wanting-to-keep-things-as-they-were feelings creates an opening to understand pain.

Focussing on the negative impact of pain makes me suffer more. But understanding pain as a signal, an alarm bell telling me when something is wrong, can take away some of the suffering.

And then there's the fact that although I feel constant pain, I wish I could feel more pain. I want *every* part of my body to send me signals about what is going on and where. Part of my journey as someone with a spinal cord injury is understanding and accepting that the brain can no longer send signals efficiently to the parts of the body below the injury site. It means I need to find other ways to check if my body is healthy.

All of the pain I experience, minor and major, can trigger distress, misery, despair, agony, torture, and anguish. Every day I make a decision not to let pain do that. My accident had already taken too much from me, so I push through. I try not to let my pain stop me from enjoying what life with my son and family has to offer.

I have learned to manage my pain. My breath is the most incredible tool. Then there is the hot-cold pack I can use to trick my brain to focus on the hot or the cold and not the pain. Massages and physio treatments and regular strengthening and stretching exercises along with repositioning tools are useful and necessary to keep my body healthy.

Not to be forgotten is psychological pain, the acute ache that threads itself through all parts of my body. When I experience the pain associated with my losses, I can focus on it and have more loss, therefore more pain, or I can tune in to the joyful moments I spend with my loved ones.

Everything changes. Nothing is permanent. Joy happens. Pain happens. And then there's more joy.

ELEVEN
PULLING FOCUS

After attending that Halifax conference, my parents and Thomas and I stayed in a house we'd rented for about ten days. We wanted to do all the things a two-year-old boy would love to do, so we spent a lot of time at the beach. My dad had found an area that was fairly well adapted for us to go to and that I could sort of navigate in my wheelchair.

What "fairly well adapted" meant was that, from the road, there were stairs that were wide enough for my parents to hoist me up one step at a time, with a large enough platform at the top of the sand dunes that then led to another series of steps. We had figured that I could either stay on top of the platform to watch Thomas and my parents play in the sand and run into the water, or my parents would bring me down step by step and then push me in the dry sand (extremely hard to do on wheels) to a place where I could transfer myself onto a towel on the sand. This way I could enjoy making sandcastles with Thomas.

The first day we did all this, everyone on the beach watched us. It was if we were animals in a zoo—or animals that had escaped from a zoo. They'd watch while trying not to be too obvious, yet with a complete inability to look away. To our left was a family of four—parents and two daughters about ten and twelve years old. There were more mature ladies sunbathing, some on the sand and others on their inflatable mattresses in the water. I guess I was looking too, looking at who was looking at us, because I noticed in one family there was a man who was incredibly muscular. In my own looking at the people looking at me, I decided the people I saw represented the usual crowd.

I played with Thomas and, when he wanted to go in the water, my parents took him in. We stayed around three or four hours, having fun with Thomas, but always with those eyes on us.

We returned to the same spot the next day. Again, those same eyes were on us as we claimed our space on the beach. This time though, the youngest of the two girls came over to us with her dad. She asked if she could play with Thomas, and offered to take him to splash in the shallows. I kindly accepted as I knew this would give my parents a much needed break. This little girl spent time building castles with Thomas and ran around playing tag with him. He loved it. When we were ready to leave, her dad offered to help us on the stairs and all the way to the car. This allowed my mom to gather all our stuff, and hold Thomas's hand. When that was done, we parted ways, but not until the man made a promise to be there next time to help out.

When we went back the third time, that father already had his eyes on the stairs. He was not watching us but watching for us. As soon as he saw us, his daughter came to get Thomas, liberating my mom. As he was about to help my dad get me down the stairs, the muscular man I'd seen before jumped in. I was carried like Cleopatra by these two beautiful men to the spot that had become ours. Those eyes were no longer watching us like animals; they were inspired by our courage and tenacity. And we inspired each other with creativity and the love and kindness we showed each other.

That day, I wanted to swim, but had no idea how I'd get to the water. My parents had thought of bringing a bedsheet onto which I could transfer, and they could then carry me into the water. Again, we carried out our plan with eyes on us. But I didn't care as I got to swim in the sea.

When we arrived on our fourth day, our routine and everyone's role had been consolidated. The young girl took care of Thomas, the men carried me, and my parents brought our things to our official spot. We were greeted by smiles and not by staring eyes. Even the quietest of spectators, those more mature women, came to us to offer me one of their inflatable mattresses. They had figured out that it would be easier and safer for me to float on one versus be carried out with a white sheet.

I could have ended my story focussing on those eyes that stared. I could have told my parents, after the first day, not to come back to that place where people saw me as a circus animal rather than a person like them. But I didn't. And in changing our own perspective on who these people were, we helped change their perspective on who we were. We were all learning about each other, adjusting to an opportunity to have a wider perspective. By the end of the week, we were just another family going on the beach to have a fun time.

My accident affected more than just me. My accident had an impact on my parents, sister, friends, and my son. But more than that, my desire and drive to continue living and participating in my son's activities and in my community affected everyone around me, including encounters with those I'd not met before.

And I do mean it had a positive impact. When strangers are sensitized to the fact that parents with disabilities exist, that they want to partake in life like any other person, that parents with disabilities need adaptations to help, then life for all improves.

On that beach in Halifax, everyone saw that a person in a wheelchair has the same aspirations as others. They had also learned about our story and how disability is something that can happen to anyone. Which means it could have happened to them. In return, it showed me how, deep down, most people are kind and want to help but sometimes just don't know how.

Many times I have heard those with a disability say how they hate when an able-bodied person asks if they need help. Some interpret that as belittlement or being less-than. But my experience has been different. I see it as people being kind and trying to reach out; at a minimum, they are acknowledging my presence which, to me, is a good thing.

Do we still have to educate everyone on the rights of people with disabilities? Yes. But we need to understand people are willing to learn and adjust; learning can be formal, or it can be situational, like at the beach.

To gain perspective, I had to use the camera in my mind's eye in that I had to choose which lens to use, and to think about how to frame each scenario. As I pull focus, changing focal length to bring new elements into sharp view, I needed to pause until there was clarity in the frame. Only then could I press the button to capture the image.

As I became a better photographer—observer—I could choose how to focus on the subject of my life and life in general. I got to choose the shutter speed, the exposure, the subject, what to blur, and what to bring into focus.

My accident taught me to slow down. We all know what photographs look like when we snap the image while we're moving. At first I didn't listen. Mental health issues got me to a place where I *had* to prioritize and set boundaries for myself.

I had known a sense of slowing down when I had my near-death experience in the accident. It was like a high-speed train that had been commanded to halt, then crawled along the tracks. The slowing down made me aware of my inner struggles and also gave me time to focus on what needed mending. As a recovering Speedy Gonzales, I could see great value in slowing down. Disability did that for me.

When you run all the time, the scenery becomes blurry. You go by so fast that you don't get to appreciate everything you pass. Instead of trying to keep up with everybody (which I couldn't do anymore—and who was I—who is anyone?—to judge how fast or slow someone else's pace is?), I needed to appreciate that paraplegia brought with it clarity. The scenes came into focus, the close-up of flowers, right to the incredible centre; the tree-lined streets from the end of the road; a wide view from the top of a hill to see the amazing valley below.

When I did this, opportunities I wouldn't have seen before appeared before my eyes. Opportunities that helped me build my resilience. Opportunities to grow. Opportunities to learn.

Yes, I wished I could walk. Yes, I wished my life was different. But those thoughts stopped me from doing what I desired the most in life. It was better, healthier, and more productive to change the settings.

Rolling Forward with New Focus

In changing our own perspective on who others are, we help change their perspective on who we are.

Focus—whether through the lens of a camera, or through the lens of our heart—allows us to capture all the beauty around us. It highlights the silver linings. These moments, when everything slowed down, when I reflected on what the present moment gave me, I could see, and I still can see, how what I experienced at those moments was a gift. I got to bear witness to the most beautiful form of humanness, and I was able to notice how precious that was. Those moments showed me that when we can pay attention to the little things, we find the silver linings.

I could wallow in misery because my car hit black ice that January morning, or I could marvel at the fact I survived. I could be angry that I lost my ability to move or feel anything below my armpits, or I could feel blessed that I am here to witness my son grow.

My silver linings are composed of all those moments I would have missed if I had died.

TWELVE
HEAD ABOVE WATER

Can a person be grateful for a shower? Yes.

After the accident, even though I was in pain, I was revived as water ran through my hair during my first shower in over a month. I had taken for granted the pleasure and luxury associated with what had been a daily routine.

Being under that stream of water reminded me of how lucky we are to have running water, even. The feeling of each of these drops of water on our skin, how invigorating the smell and lather of soap is, how having our hair scrubbed and washed with shampoo gets us ready to face the world. Feeling and being clean is amazing. I'd been taking it for granted.

That day, February 3, 2012, I was grateful for the actual shower —water, soap, cleansing—and also for the nurse who took her time and stayed longer to allow me to feel like a human again.

Allowing myself to touch and express gratitude to that nurse for that shower took me past the shower, past the nurse, to those who manufactured the shampoo, the truck drivers who transported it to the store, the truck driver's truck, the mechanic, the people who made the road, the cashier who placed it in a bag… and so on in never-ending tentacles of gratefulness.

The first ten days following my accident, as I was slowly grasping what had happened and what it meant, a great team of doctors, nurses, and *préposés* (nursing aids) were taking care of my body and, in doing so, my soul. I will always be grateful to them.

Being grateful and expressing gratitude to others for their kindness is both part of the point and not the point. I can be grateful because people are nice to me, and since I don't think I deserve the attention and support they offer me, I feel the need to thank them. Or I can learn to be grateful for the things that are given or offered to me because I deserve them. Although feeling gratitude had always been easy for me, I needed to learn to connect it to knowing I was deserving.

Feeling grateful is as easy as it is hard.

Looking at life with gratitude made me focus on the good and the beautiful things that had happened every single day. It made me mindful of what was great even when I was surrounded by challenges. It made me pause and focus. When I expressed my gratitude, it made me feel better by highlighting their value and contribution to the world.

Rehabilitation is fuelled by people. Great people, all kinds of people, devoted people with encouraging smiles and firm yet gentle hands. Each rehabilitation specialist fit into a piece of a larger puzzle. Every day, each person demonstrated their capacity to see beyond my limitations. Through their kindness, generosity, and heart, rehabilitation allowed me, and others like me, to regain and reconstruct our wings. Those people—professionals and friends—who improve our quality of life at a time when we don't feel we have any quality of life—are the catalyst to renewing a sense of gratitude. It is difficult not to be grateful for—and to—those who are there to help.

There were many reasons I had to be grateful from the beginning: from the hospital staff in the acute phase, to stage two staff in the rehabilitation process and, finally, to stage three staff whose focus was on reinsertion into normal life. In each phase, I wrote letters to show my gratitude to everyone who went beyond, whose dedication to my recovery was paramount.

The first letter I wrote was the one I mentioned previously, ten days after the accident, to the doctor who had a child the same age as Thomas.

The gratitude I felt for the professionals on this intensive care unit is not something I can describe or explain. It is beyond anything I had seen in my life.

And so, in remembering the extraordinary care I had received in the acute phase, I also wrote a letter thanking them for sustaining my life and uplifting my soul when all I'd wanted to do—at that time—was curl up in a ball and die. I thanked them for their compassion and for the respect and dignity they allowed me. They were the first ones who showed me that I had value.

In phase two, also called intensive rehabilitation, I wrote another letter to the team caring for me. But I also kept retelling the story of my first intervention plan meeting.

Prior to my accident, I taught many future healthcare workers how to craft intervention plans. I knew how intervention plans were done and I also knew quite well how they should be done. With my accident, I got to see how it was done from a patient's point of view. I got to sit at the head of the table to chair my own intervention plan meeting. I experienced how a group of seven professionals could come together and offer interventions geared toward the goal I wanted to achieve the most: to be mom to Thomas.

As we progressed through each intervention phase, the goal had to be clarified. And at the end, the goal was stripped to its most simple form: *to connect with my son*. I learned new ways to connect, interact, and raise an eighteen-month-old, then a twenty-month-old, twenty-two-month-old, then a two-year-old, three-, four-, and five-year-old. This objective was ongoing, adaptable, and customized to the reality my son brought to the situation.

Out of all the intervention plans I had seen and participated in, this was, by far, the best.

After phase two, there was a little pause in my rehabilitation. A pause to allow me to return home. Although it was a great feeling to be home, my house had become such a mess that it was hard to be grateful. Since the bedrooms were upstairs, I slept in the living room or the dining room with some of my *stuff* (clothes, mail, insurance papers) piled anywhere and everywhere. I was still grateful for being close to Thomas and for having my mom around—she slept over. I would get to feed him, prepare his meals, even get him dressed, and prepare him for daycare. Doing those mom tasks made me happy to have survived the accident.

Phase three of my rehabilitation meant learning more skills. External rehabilitation meant I had to learn within my environment. This was where I received a lot of help to fight my fear of driving, help regarding how my parenting could be adapted, and support in my plan to go back to work (even if they thought it would be too much for me).

I became beyond excited for, and happy when, I was able to move into my *new* adapted house—March 2013. For the first time in a little more than fourteen months, I was able to tuck my son into his *new* bed (no more crib), in our new house. I thanked all the professionals who made this possible, and wrote pages of gratitude in my journal.

Team Phase Three and I remodelled and created new solutions: like when I wanted to learn to swim safely around Thomas. In order to do that, my kinesiologist (physical therapist) had searched and found tools to help me float. In 2016, she found a belt that helped me swim in the beautiful Pacific Ocean off the shores of Hawaii. And that led to more gratitude as it became key in helping me save my son.

Thomas had become more confident in the water. He and I were talking while swimming in the ocean—my mom was floating nearby. As I was chatting with Thomas, I turned my head for a moment to see how far away my mom was. When I turned back I realized Thomas's feet were not touching the sea-bed anymore. He started to panic. I called out to my mom but she had floated far enough away that she didn't immediately understand me. I knew I had to do something to rescue him, so I grabbed onto him. Then I realized that his weight, added to mine, challenged my buoyancy level and balance and I was going to go under.

I prepared myself to go under, to swallow and even to breathe in seawater, if that's what it was going to take to keep my son's head above water. But thankfully, the physical therapist had taken into consideration my weight and that of my son. I bobbed and dipped and then we righted again. My mom saw we needed help and as she reached us, the incident was over as quickly as it began.

I was overflowing with gratitude.

Rolling Forward with Gratitude

Gratitude could only take root once I embraced how fortunate I was to be here, that every moment is a gift-wrapped package of newness.

For me, it took my thinking about what I would have missed out on if I had not survived, things my cousin, Sylvia, would not have wanted to miss.

My wheelchair gives me opportunities to roam around and go about my life. Without it, I would be in bed, stuck in my room.

Expressing gratitude allowed me to notice the good, keep noticing the good, and to put in place a practice that meant good thoughts brought more good thoughts, and so on. It's like when you buy a red car, and suddenly everyone seems to have a red car. Whatever we focus on multiplies. Expands. In essence, when we are thankful for one thing, then a second, we begin cultivating a whole garden of things we are thankful for and appreciate.

Every moment of gratitude contains a seed of energy, happiness, and hope. When I express gratitude, it promotes the ability to be aware of the positive within. Gratitude practices modify biochemistry and brain structures to focus more and more on positives. It creates an upward spiral, and I can manage stressful events better.

Gratitude gave me respite in a world that had gotten pretty dark. It was also my way to give back or pay it forward to the people who lifted me up when I was down.

THIRTEEN

HEROES AND SHEROES

I was back in that moment before impact,
his giggles in my ears. *Let me live.*

As parents, we often have to be reminded of how strong we are. As moms on wheels, especially when we have only just acquired our wheels, we really need to hear—and believe—how strong we are.

Because we are. Strong.

We're doing life every moment. We're doing life right now. We should be proud because what we're doing is actually amazing. When we can admit—even a tiny bit—that we are incredible, doubt begins to slip away and, along with it, so fades shame and all the chilling and aggressive inner critics that allow shame to hold us back.

Our perception of the situations of others is skewed. We often see everyone else's successes, but not the path they took to get there. For that reason, we think they've had it easy, and we wonder why we are not having it easy. The thing is, if we asked them about their journey, their stories would also be filled with missteps and failures and struggle.

Just as some of our heroes and sheroes and mentors, who moved mountains to be who and where they are, those of us who do not yet see ourselves as sheroes of our own lives can be courageous change-makers too.

I was thirty-four years old when I was in that car accident. As I lay there, I directed myself to stay calm, to trust that the first responders were doing everything in their power to save me.

Which was miraculous. Me, the control junky, relinquish control? But I did. I relinquished control in a situation where others were definitely better equipped to do a good job. Facing a life-changing situation with my head held as high as I could, considering the circumstances, I was letting others help me, show me, teach me. At thirty-four, I was learning everything again. Starting in those moments after impact, I was being brave.

During rehabilitation, fear was my constant emotion. But courage is when we roll forward *despite* the fear. Every first, every new movement, every transfer needed to be taken and performed with an incredible amount of courage.

Like the time the occupational therapist asked me to pick up a box of Kleenex he'd placed on the floor.

I cried. I couldn't stop sobbing. I wanted to hit him. I wanted to swear at him. The feeling of bending down over my legs, without feeling my feet, brought vivid memories of the time I rappelled down from a sixty-foot cliff over the Blue Mountains two hours south of Sydney, Australia: the sensation of bending and leaning over an empty space, the terror of potentially falling into nothingness. I was terrified. The only possible response to his request and to those tears was picking up the box of Kleenex. I hated him for asking me to do this and I am eternally grateful he did, because this was a moment that symbolized my determination, my courage, for every other small and not-so-small request to come in rehab and beyond.

I had been rolling forward for a while, adjusting to the emotional and physical changes of my renarrated life, while still renarrating it—do we ever stop?—when my sister came to town for Christmas.

There was a new Disney movie playing at the theatre so, in my role of auntie, I decided to take her children and my son to the movies. The three older kids already knew the rules as I had coached them many times. But it was the first time my niece, Alexandra, was coming with me. I explained, "Alex, if you come with us, there are some very clear rules we all follow to make sure everyone is safe."

The kids knew to wait in the car until I was in my wheelchair. Then they followed the plan that, once I was in the chair, they'd get out and glue themselves to the car, then hold on to my hand, or scarf, or bag—something that is attached to me. They also knew that if, at any time, I decided it was unsafe, we would return home. No movie. Safety first. Always.

As we arrived, everything went as planned. Every child listened and followed the rules.

Then the juggling act began as I realized the following: I needed to have four seats near the spot reserved for people with disabilities—for wheelchairs. Then, I would need a booster seat for Alex. I'd also need to carry drinks and popcorn for everyone. I had not thought that through. Oh, and we all had glasses to wear as it was a 3D movie.

I ordered the four popcorns and drinks and I sent two of the oldest, nine and ten years old, to carry the popcorn and save the seats. The third eldest, eight, helped me get the booster seat and carried it.

I was proud of myself. After dispatching everyone to their assigned tasks, Alex said, "Tata, I have to go pee." At that moment, feeling as if I was juggling eight balls in the air, I had to decide: bring the third eldest to the other two who were waiting in the theatre, or bring the third eldest along with Alex and me to the bathroom? For a split second I feared this would tip me past the point of being able to masterfully juggle it all.

But we worked it out. We had fun.

Later, I told my sister about it, thinking she'd be proud of me. "This happens to all mommies who bring a few kids to the movies."

My being on wheels was an irrelevant detail.

Little acts of courage accumulated over time. I drove to the movies. There had been a time when I said I'd never get in a car again, ever. And never drive. But I had. There was a time when I couldn't imagine what it would take to go somewhere with my son but, little by little, I'd built the skills to take four kids to the movies. At the movies, little by little—with safety in mind—I adjusted our plans and did not give up. Then I discovered that the challenges I faced, and solutions I came up with, are those faced by all moms.

Being a parent is a massive act of courage and requires many acts of bravery.

Maybe I was brave for having survived. Maybe I was brave for having adapted to my new life circumstances. Maybe courage helped me face all those struggles with my dignity (mostly) intact. Maybe I needed to recognize my efforts and give myself a pat on the back for a job well done.

Regardless, I was uncomfortable with words that painted me a shero—brave, courageous, powerful, superwoman. What others might describe as bravery, I saw as love: love of learning (going on another camping trip, travelling, living abroad, learning about spinal cord injury) and love for others. Partly it was my humble Canadian-ness, partly I just didn't at first see myself as brave. I didn't believe in me.

The bigger the fear, the greater the courage.
Brava all of us moms on wheels.
Brava you.
Say it!
Brava me, dammit.
Brava you courageous, valiant, warrior of a human!

Bravery is a strength we all have. In my situation, my bravery showed up as knowing when to ask for help, advocating for parents with disabilities as an all-inclusive group, calling out systemic discrimination, and working to help keep the government account-able to their ratification of the UN Convention on the Rights of Persons with Disabilities.

And it showed up when I decided to share details of my struggles and how I overcame them. Sharing, with vulnerability and authenticity, in speaking competitions and right here on these pages.

Recognizing I can be brave is empowering as it means I don't let things happen *to* me. I can be an agent of change who takes risks and grows. The more I use bravery, the more I learn to cope more efficiently and effectively when challenged.

The more confident I feel, the more I will try something new, like taking four children to the movies. The more I am able to challenge myself, despite fear and anxiety, the more I can reach out and demonstrate resilience.

Each of us moms on wheels is brave as we live with a disability, as we face chronic pain, as we deal with the challenges of the day-to-day, and we do it all in a world heavily prejudiced against those with disabilities.

And each of us moms on wheels is courageous in accepting what is.

For all of us moms on wheels, redefining what has happened, reframing the impact certain events have had on our lives, and making incremental moves toward realistic goals are each acts of bravery.

Moments of doubt and fear of failure will creep in. Bravery does not mean there are no tears. The opposite, really. We need to remind ourselves of that. Those moments are necessary for us to keep growing. We can't prevent ourselves from falling or tipping, but we can get up again. Or crawl if necessary.

This is the biggest brave: to learn to be brave with ourselves, despite, and in acceptance of, our vulnerabilities. Regardless of how open we are in front of others, the tears have a time and place —and when we cry with pride and bravery, instead of shame, is the most magnificent brave of all. Those tears—our tears shed that way—are signs that we dare, that we push through the fear and roll forward with strength, with determination, and for ourselves, so that we create legacy for our children. And so we be brave. Then we be brave again. And again.

FOURTEEN
FLAWED PREMISE

Many fiercely independent people miss out on the beauty of reciprocation and operate from the flawed premise that receiving assistance exposes their weaknesses and makes them less.

When we realize that asking for help is a strength and not a weakness, life flows more smoothly. But it is hard to convince stubbornly autonomous individuals that the giving and receiving of help is a glorious exchange that fertilizes our growth and creates a healthy balance.

A cup of milk here. An egg there. A school pick-up one afternoon. A "can you water my plants while I'm away?" We recognize these requests as neighbourly. They are the catalyst for connection.

There is this story that's been around on social media—unattributed—about a family who had a lot (of stuff) and their neighbours who did not have a lot (of stuff). One day, the mom of the have-a-lot-of-stuff family asked her child to go over to the neighbour's and ask for a teaspoon of salt. The child was confused, pointing out they had plenty of salt in the saltshaker. The mom explained to the child that asking for something once in a while, something they knew the person would have and not miss, was a way to encourage others to ask for things or help.

I'd add to that story and say it's also a way to signal to anyone who might view themselves as a have-not that someone else sees them as having enough to ask. It's a small act of kindness.

The fact is that strong people ask for help.

When something blows up our lives, it is difficult to handle the fallout by ourselves. And it's equally difficult to know how to ask for help. We forget that people genuinely want to help and as much as we don't know how to ask, they don't know how to offer. They don't know what we need.

This is why it is okay—more than okay—to ask for specifically what you need. It's not bossy or demanding to be direct and explain what you need. If your friend was going through a crisis and you were asked to prepare food for her family, wouldn't you want to have a list of likes, dislikes, and allergies?

After my accident, you already know I saw myself as drastically different. I felt needy and couldn't fathom that it was okay for me to ask for help. All my life I had pursued a fierce independence. While I still needed to be valued, understood, seen, recognized, loved, and cared for, I felt I was exposing and then imposing my limitations on my loved ones. I knew how to give help—but I had no idea how to receive it gracefully and graciously.

I felt like a burden and hated needing so much from everyone. In a way, it's what motivated me to work so hard in my physical and occupational therapy sessions—though another motivator was to be able to parent—and eventually, when I renarrated my life, it meant I would be able to resume helping others in my professional life.

But it was hard for me to break the limiting belief that while giving help was strong, receiving help was weak. At least when it concerned me.

Among my biggest challenges was to overcome the resistance I had to being vulnerable. I thought if I let my vulnerabilities show through, the whole dam would break and everything I was feeling was going to flood my street, neighbourhood, and my entire city. Walls would fall down and I'd be powerless to stop it.

But reality kept catching up to me: I needed help. And if I didn't learn to accept it—fast—my son would be the one to perish. I needed people to come along on our journey. I needed them by my side. Who knew—certainly not me at that time—that when I was asking for help I was saying that I cared? I was saying that I trusted them. I was saying that I loved them.

At first this was difficult. I needed to practice because it was a new concept for me.

Over time, I began to understand that asking for help provides opportunities for everyone to learn how to ask and offer help without disempowering the other person. Just like the mom who asked her have-not neighbour for salt. My asking for help created connections and grew relationships.

It still boggles my mind to know how many people wanted to come visit me when I was in the hospital. Although I was happy people felt compelled to wish me well, I was overwhelmed. I felt I needed to look good and be okay. To show good faith. To be strong. I didn't want to be vulnerable in front of them, as I had different levels of intimacy with everyone who showed up. Most were personal friends, but some were my work colleagues. Some were my staff—even if I sometimes went for drinks with them after a day at the office, they were still in my employ, so it was hard for me to be seen as any less than I was used to being. And I wasn't ready to accept that I could no longer be that person.

Seeing these gracious visitors while wearing a blue gown tied only by three little strings in the back was embarrassing. And I also felt compelled to comfort some of them or convince them that life would be okay for me. There were even times I felt I needed to reassure them that their life would stay the same, even though I didn't yet know what the accident would do to my life or their place in it.

Those visits took their toll. They forced me to reflect on the person I would no longer be. I was disappointed—for them and for me.

So, I asked that only a select few be allowed to visit, and only at certain times. If Thomas was with me, he was my priority. This meant I wanted no other visitors when I was with him. That was our sacred time. He needed uninterrupted time with me and I with him.

Phone calls were also screened or ignored. Sometimes, I was physically incapable of picking up the phone that was beside my hospital bed because moving and twisting my body to reach the two or three feet meant something entirely different than before. When I did pick up, or when my mom picked up for me, I hated talking on the phone because I'd get the thousand-question conversation and, when that one was over, the next conversation would be the same. "How are you doing? What did the doctor say?" All I wanted was to hear about them and their normal lives, but no one wants to share the seemingly mundane when a crisis has taken place.

Yet the mundane is what I wanted to hear about. Needed to hear about.

I didn't want to have to go over what happened, or the prognosis, or recount how things were for my parents or me, or how Thomas was going to be affected. Yet I understood everyone's need to connect with me. I just didn't know how to put it all together to streamline conversation and conserve my energy.

Until my friend-boss-mentor showed up, excited, with a package. The staff had collected money to purchase an iPad complete with a SIM card so that I could stay connected to everyone online. One post on Facebook with news and everyone could be informed. They could answer back, post funny emojis, or hearts, or even inappropriate comments if they thought that would help, and I could review their reactions without feeling pressure to respond if I wasn't up to it. Facebook became my way to stay connected, to feel like I still belonged here on this earth, without having to fake it or look good. It was just what I needed.

Online, I was able to ask for what I needed when I needed it. Months later, when I returned home and saw how messy my backyard was, I posted a request for help to clean it up and make it toddler-proof. About fifty people came to help us that day.

The iPad allowed me to connect with my favourite person in the whole wide world: my son. Using FaceTime or Skype, me in hospital or rehab, Thomas at home with my mom, we could eat breakfast together, and do Thomas's evening routine together. I saw him build his first snowman and I was "with" him the first morning he went to his new daycare. I could be with Thomas and he could see I was still with him.

Some of my girlfriends would come regularly to the hospital and feed me home-cooked meals that they'd prepared. Others went directly to my house to drop off meals for my parents, knowing they were taking on more responsibility for Thomas than before. My boss arranged for her nanny to help care for my son, even though her own son had started school. Knowing that each and every one of them was there made a huge difference in my life and in my well-being. I didn't have to worry or stew so much as I knew people—mainly my parents—were taking care of those responsibilities. And I didn't have to worry as much about my parents when I knew that other people, at times, were also taking care of them.

My aunt was in my room every morning to help with post-waking routines. My mom would bring Thomas every day and return after supper every evening to help me brush my teeth and make sure I was tired enough to fall asleep after she left—so that I wouldn't be scared to be alone. I kept saying I didn't need her to come back every day after bringing Thomas but, the reality was, I really did. And she knew it. I didn't know what I needed but my mom and my aunt and my friends and colleagues did. And they were right.

Asking for help is only the first part. We have to learn to accept it when it is offered and to respond gracefully. We have to know we deserve that help. The journey of my asking and accepting expanded over time, like ripples in a pond.

My first postaccident international trip—from Montreal, to Paris, to Helsinki, to Turku—took place about sixteen months postaccident. I was so proud I could travel on my own and do my own transfers. I could transfer from my wheelchair to the airplane chair to the airplane seat, to the airplane chair, to the transporter chair, to a transporter wheelchair, to an airport wheelchair—so many transfers! Every time I was asked to change seats I did, but my pride was making my shoulders hurt.

So, when the *next* guy at the next airport informed me that my wheelchair was waiting for me somewhere else and that he needed to take back the chair I was currently sitting on until *another* guy would come to pick me up in *yet another* chair, I decided enough was enough. "Stop," I said. "You want me to transfer yet again? After a night in a plane and knowing that I have two other flights and a transfer to my hotel? Okay, no problem." Then with a huge smile, I lifted my arms up toward him and said, "If you want me to transfer into another seat, you carry me!"

He did. And so did the next guy and the next for the rest of that trip. My overall energy and my shoulders' health were and are more important than my pride.

If I need help, I now know to ask for it. Even better, I now know to plan for help ahead of time.

Shit happens. Why should I—or any of us moms on wheels be exempt? Metaphorical shitty situations happen to all of us. Few have to deal with the literal shitty situation.

But I did. Like the day my nurse thought of giving me a laxative to help disimpact me—yes, there were (and are) numerous times I was full of shit. LOL. What the nurse couldn't know is that lactulose would have a powerful effect on me. It worked so well that an explosion and overflow happened.

I was so ashamed, I wanted to cry. Yet my nurse kept laughing. She could not stop. She explained between bursts of laughter that she had been wrong to give me lactulose, laughing about how *she* now had to clean up *her* mess.

After more than twenty months of not seeing each other (thank you, COVID-19), my mom, Thomas, and I finally got to spend some time with my sister and her family. We decided I'd rent an adapted room at the hotel that I'm used to so that my mom could spend time relaxing and have much-needed time with her other daughter. I decided I'd have the three older kids, including my son, with me in my room. I had one bed, two kids shared the other bed, and the third slept in a cot beside them. I'd travelled with them before so I knew they were great at occupying themselves and following directions, and were independent in all their self-care routines.

I had just gotten dressed in my pyjamas and transferred into my bed. I was about to invite the kids back into the room when I realized I was dangerously close to having a shitty catastrophe.

Murphy's Law… isn't it? Having practiced mindfulness for almost two years by then, I see the shame come through in my head. I see the little girl desperately wanting to ask for her mom. But in my head was also the grown-up woman who knew she could do it. I called the kids back into the room and told them I had an issue and needed to take care of myself. I then told them what my expectations were, that I needed to count on them because I could not check on them, I would simply check on them by texting from the bathroom.

I managed to get in the bathroom, go about my business, shower and go back to bed after the kids were asleep. For the first time since my accident, I felt like "I got it." Despite having had another unfortunate incident, I didn't feel any shame or guilt or frustration. I did what I had to do, and I moved on.

When shit happens and our focus is on surviving, it makes it easier on us, or whoever has to substitute for us, if some resources are already in place. Knowing something could happen helps us prepare for if or when that something does happen. We can't have everything organized for every just-in-case, but we can have the basics in place.

FIFTEEN
GRUNTS AND GRIT

When I was a teenager, I would often go and hang out in Sylvia's bedroom. Since my aunt and uncle's house was in between my school and my house, it was easy for me to stop by when I felt like it. In her room was a poster of a beautiful, majestic swan, with text underneath that read:

TO TRY IS THE BEST WAY TO SUCCEED

I would stare at that poster every time, mesmerized by its message. Believing in this quote led me to stand a whole day as backup in case there was an extra space for cadet camp (which there was, and I got to go twice to camp that summer). It influenced me to get into my PhD program when I didn't have the marks. I found the back door, a way to show that I had grit, which the professors admired—it was to their advantage to accept a student they knew had the drive to graduate.

I worked hard and didn't let go of my dreams. I took opportunities and showed up with my work ethic. I had been hired as a research assistant. My contract gave me sixty hours over two weeks to enter the data from piles of questionnaires. I managed to finish it all in thirty-five hours. As I told the professor I was done, he was impressed, not only by my capacity to work hard but also to be honest—there was a risk I'd only get paid for thirty-five hours and not sixty. So he gave me more complicated work. As I kept working, the contracts kept coming, until he suggested I apply for a research position under his supervision.

Perseverance and determination also served me well as I was doing my PhD, conducting my interviews while juggling work contracts and taking courses. During my worst year, I was working close to ninety hours per week: Monday to Thursday fourteen hours per day, Friday eight, Saturday and Sunday twelve hours each. Never giving up.

Of course, that might have been past grit, into ridiculousness, and on the road to burnout.

February 2, 2012, was a day when I regained some control over my life. After four weeks of being in a hospital gown, I got to wear clothes. Real clothes! Just being asked to get dressed was the first step. It felt marvellous to be up, as though I was ready for work, presentable in front of strangers. I felt ready to be out and about in the community.

I had felt ready to saddle up and ride for days. In the hospital, my recovery had progressed enough and the patient-staff ratio was so high that I was pretty much left alone. The promise of physical work was exhilarating. Getting dressed and moving to a rehabilitation centre was a big deal.

Every pothole on the drive from the hospital to the rehabilitation centre brought excruciating pain—perhaps a sign of things to come. Once we arrived, the driver of the adapted van said, "Here, they make miracles—if you work hard enough." I figured I could pursue my own miracle. After all, working hard was something I could do. I didn't yet understand that miracles happen on their own time, on their own terms, and they write their own definition. On that day, me walking again was the miracle I wanted to work for. I didn't yet conceive that my miracle might be being alive, being healthy, and being here to raise Thomas, or even the amazing staff I was about to meet.

I was rapidly introduced to normal things—things I'd taken for granted. Normal things that made me feel, well, normal! First, I was transferred *on* a bed, in a very nice room with windows facing the sunlight and trees. Health professionals who would help me get stronger started coming in to introduce themselves. It was nice to know who would be supporting me as the whole concept of rehabilitation was in a way, ironically, foreign to me. I got cleaned up and dressed in gym clothes and went for my first physio treatment.

That first introduction to the rehabilitation process shocked me into action.

Since my accident, each transfer was done via a lift of some sort or with the help of two human beings. I'd be hoisted into the air and transferred from my bed to my wheelchair or from the chair to the bed. This was keeping me dependent upon the availability of a mechanical lift and two certified people.

But my physiotherapist set the tone for our relationship on that first session when he asked me to do my own transfer—from my chair to the physio table and without a board. Scary! I didn't yet know how to stay stable while in a sitting position, I didn't know if my arm muscles were strong enough to carry my body weight as my back muscles shifted me onto the other surface. *Saddle up!* I had no idea if I could do this, but my physiotherapist did. His confidence gave me no choice: I had to believe I would land on the bed. And I did.

When he asked me to do pull ups a few days later, I was ready to work on my arm and shoulder muscles. My goal: thirty pull-ups, nonstop. He was there encouraging me, counting with me. I was smiling. As we closed in on thirty pull-ups he announced he wanted ten more. I told him off, still smiling, then said, "No problem." I kept counting, but when I was close to forty, he said I still looked fresh and to keep going, maybe to fifty. I made a few jokes, swore at him mostly, and headed to fifty. At forty-eight he told me that because I was still smiling, I was good to go to seventy.

I started to grunt, couldn't speak anymore, but carried on. Near seventy he asked for ten more for good luck. We got to eighty, which he quickly said was way too close to one hundred to stop. At that point I could no longer speak so kept counting in my head through to the magic number and just as I was on one hundred he called out for one more, just because. I finished with one hundred and one under my belt. I was focussed on the task at hand. In my bubble. I was productive. I was persevering.

I persevered every day in rehab. The work was concrete, tangible, and it felt good! Because it took all my concentration and my willpower was strong, nothing else mattered at that point. The pain, the loss, the hurt that followed my accident were invisible. In those moments at physio, I was untouchable! It gave me power, recharged my batteries, made me feel alive. And it felt… great! It also helped give purpose to the time I was away from Thomas.

I trusted my physiotherapist. I told him my goal was to walk again. He took that as evidence of my drive to work hard. And as he pushed me to my limits, he also helped me understand that the spine is not like skin or bones: it does not grow back or repair itself. Still he motivated me to thrive knowing things were different. He pushed me to my limits without pushing me over the edge.

Just enough for me to get a little bit stronger than last time, despite the pain. Because he knew I could, I knew I could. I was going to train as hard as I possibly could to regain as much control as I could over my body. And I knew I needed to do what my physio said so that I could be a mother to Thomas.

Rolling Forward with Perseverance in Balance

Perseverance is required for success—and balance is required for successful and healthy outcomes.

Perseverance had always been a part of my makeup. Dealing with my spinal cord injury was a little different, and it took my mental crash to force me to figure out that not only do I need to keep going, I also need to respect and move at my new pace. In my case, I needed to incorporate my fears and posttraumatic responses and deal with them as they were also part of my rehabilitation process. I needed to accept that the journey toward acceptance might be a long one and that instead of looking too far ahead into the future, I just needed to focus on the task at hand.

Today, the message from Sylvia's poster inspires me to keep trying, yes, but to do so in a way that is balanced, respectful of the reality I'm living.

SIXTEEN

ARE YOU SURE, LITTLE LADY?

I learned to release humour, sometimes a rather dark humour, and it alleviated the heaviness of difficult times—for me and for those around me.

Without humour, I know I would not have survived my first few years postaccident. My mom wouldn't have either.

My mom was the person who was the closest to me in the first few years. She was the one holding down the fort at home, with the support of my dad of course. She was also my personal assistant in some regards. When bad things, like incontinence, happened to me, they happened to her. And when you have to enter the most intimate world of your grown-up daughter as she had to, laughing through it was much better than the alternative. Crying would only have made it worse.

Humour certainly served my mom and I well, as it unified us in times where it could have divided us due to shame or guilt. Humour was an essential ingredient of our common resilience, especially each time we were faced with challenging situations, or when we felt despair creeping in. It took out the scary, the shameful, the disgusting, the awkward, the overwhelming—all those negative emotions that can weigh us down. Humour enhanced the love we have for each other, redefined our acts of kindness, and made us see who we were and are in the truest form of human-hood. It certainly helped me gain a different, more playful, more positive perspective on the cards I'd been dealt in my life.

Exercising my humour muscles and embracing the silly gave me tools to combat uncertainty. Difficult times were not as serious or perceived as permanent. With humour, we were reminded that tough times would pass. It also was associated with a different memory-making process: we later remembered the laughter and not the horrid event we were laughing about. And that is powerful.

Incorporating humour in some situations after my accident took the uneasiness out of them. The best and funniest parts were people's reactions. Some preferred to ignore my comments, others would squirm uncomfortably as they laughed, a few would half-smile, and still others would burst out laughing. Using humour defused the awkwardness people had at first with me being a para-plegic or being in a wheelchair. When we laughed about it, I stopped being a person to pity. When I used humour it gave others permission to openly talk about the elephant in the room: my chair, my accident, my spinal cord injury.

It had been weeks since my accident and my legs were a hairy mess. As nurses and nurses' aides came into my room, my mom blurted, in a serious tone and with a pinch of jealousy, "You are one lucky lady! Now you can wax without ever feeling pain!"

On weekends, Thomas and I regularly ate breakfast in my bed. One morning, Thomas arrived in my bedroom with his box of cereal, ready to eat. But I was already in the midst of transferring into my chair.

"No, Thomas! Today we eat breakfast at the table."

Thomas was visibly sad about this news. "Why, Mom?"

"Well, because this morning you play hockey, and I am already up." We were speaking in French, and so the phrase was *je suis debout* or "I am standing."

Thomas started laughing. "You are not standing, Mom... you are in a wheelchair!" Then he walked to the kitchen.

At work, I would roll from one meeting to the next, which was sometimes challenging from a punctuality perspective. Arriving a few minutes late, sometimes more, I'd serve up one of my newest excuses:

"Sorry I'm late... I had a flat tire on the way."

As I tried to ensure I scheduled enough time between meetings to minimize my lateness, I'd say, "Sorry, I can't meet tomorrow morning, I have an appointment to put my winter tires on."

On landing at the airport in Vienna, there was meant to be an adapted taxi to bring us to our hotel. Instead, we found a very nice driver who had a van. A van with no other way to get in than to jump in, which happened to be a bit difficult for someone like me. Not knowing the place and wanting to get to the hotel in a timely manner, my mom and I were faced with only one solution: have that really nice driver grab my ass to hoist me up! I could have cried. I could have yelled. I could have reacted in many different ways, but I chose to laugh it out because that option was better than any other.

Little jokes like these provided a way for me to adjust to my new reality and for me to allow others to glimpse the new reality as well. And humour was used regularly in my house, with my mom —or anyone else—who would have to take care of my body. It helped me ease my way through difficult situations.

The biggest running gag in my family, because it was too stupid to be true, happened during my rehab.

We desperately needed to find a way to adapt my parents' van as I was not able to get into their car. Modification was important so that I would not be limited to the types of activities I could do with my son. We were searching for examples.

One day, a man came to show me the van he had adapted for his wife, who had a hip injury. He'd installed a lift on the passenger side of the van. I was so excited that I even asked some of my friends from rehabilitation if they wanted to come and see how it worked as they, too, needed something to allow them to get into their vehicles.

As I came close to the lift I realized it was too high for me to transfer on it. Just a little too high.

Disappointed, I thanked him for coming—for going out of his way to be kind and helpful.

Saddened by this, this extremely determined and kind man tried different ways to lower the lift to my height, but nothing worked. Our conversation went a little like this:

Man: "Are you sure, little lady, that you can't go up on the lift?"

Me: "Yes... unfortunately, I can't lift my body this high. So, it won't work."

Man: "You know... my wife stands up to sit on it. Maybe if you got up a little, you could do it too."

Me: "Hmmm, sir, the reason I need the lift is because I cannot get up."

Man: "Okay, I understand. But I am not asking you to stand up, just to get up a little. It would work, you know... if you got up a little."

Me: "Yes... I understand. I also wish I could get up a little. If I could, I would not have asked you to come down here and I would not require this lift."

Man: "Of course, of course. Well, maybe you could just put a bit of weight on your legs and straighten them. It would help you sit on the platform."

Me: "Right. But then that would mean that I had gotten up a little like you asked me already. And, I am sorry to say (yet again) that I cannot do this."

Man: "Oh, right. That's too bad."

(Me, in my head: *Exactly, you're telling me!*)

Man: "Maybe you could get up just a little bit. It won't take much, I promise."

Me: "You know. I think you are right. Maybe I could get up just a little."

Man: "Really? You can get up a bit? Great!"

Me: "Nope. I can't get up. Not even a bit. Thank you for coming."

There were many times, in trying to be funny, that I missed the boat. And there were times when I wasn't trying to be funny but the comment would make me laugh uncontrollably.

People with careers like homicide detectives, coroners, surgeons, journalists, undertakers, plumbers, and exterminators also use humour to defuse situations they encounter. And because those situations are often dark, the humour that counterbalances the horrible is dark humour.

I learned I was capable of that humour when I was out with my best girls. It wasn't actually a night out—we were together at a wake—a serious, emotional event to celebrate someone else's life. At first, we spoke quietly, but after all the other mourners had left, we hung out and started laughing, teasing, and roasting one another.

I had planned to stay until nine-ish, but it was close to midnight when my mom texted me. "R u ok?" I texted back a "Yes," then told my friend, who was giving me a ride back home, that it was time to leave. Our conversation went something like this:

Judy: "Your mom texted?"

Me: "Yes, she is asking if I'm okay."

Judy: "What did you say?"

Me: "Well," (pretending I am texting) "Am ok, just in a ditch somewhere."

Then I looked up at Judy. "Oops! Wait, I used this once already. This is not an excuse you want to use twice."

Stupid. Insensitive. Yet when I said it, I could not stop laughing.

But this is what we do. And it's important to know this. As moms on wheels, we need to know that dark humour is a part of life. Some would say it is a life-saver in that it eases the moments. Laughter releases tension and ushers it out the door. Laughter—from looking at the ridiculous part of life's situations—invites perspective in a less analytical way than serious study.

And sometimes humour is so on the line that it is not humour, but a raw, authentic, awkward honesty that, while there is no laughter resulting, the release has the same effect.

Like the gloomy day I bought a new car. The difficult process of buying the car caused me nausea, headaches, and sleepless nights

—even though my parents did all the legwork. It took every ounce of energy to force myself to go to the car dealership to sign the papers. Once there, I only paid attention to what I needed to know in each moment—the rest of the time I took my mind to a beach and the imaginings of tropical places in order to ease the anxiety and to stop the running thoughts that plagued me.

But everyone else at the car dealership was happy I was buying a car. Happy for me… of course. Aren't people usually happy when they buy a new car? Even the lady in the financing department was ecstatic.

Lady: "Congratulations on your new car. You must be so happy. It is a great car. What colour did you choose?"

Me: "Grey, I think."

Lady: "Oh wow. The lighter grey or darker one?"

Me: "I don't know. My mom picked out the colour."

Lady: "A 2015 model. Super. Lucky you."

Me: "I guess."

Lady: "How many kilometres do you expect to drive annually?"

Me: "I don't know. Look, please just say what you have to say. Tell me what you offer, but please stop talking about how great it is for me to have a car. Last time I had one I got in a fucking accident that left me paralyzed. If you ask me, I don't care about the model, the colour, or the car itself. That's why my parents did the legwork for me. And the numbers of kilometres annually? I would love to tell you but I can't. That's because I don't want to drive any kilometres. I would like to do none. Just go through whatever you are selling because I am feeling nauseous and just want to get home."

Silence.

Lady: "Hey. So sorry."

While this was not a funny-ha-ha moment for me or for the finance person, it represents an honest communication that was an alternative to breaking down and crying my eyes out.

The types of humour range from knock-knock jokes from our kids to serious, dark, and disturbing releases of honesty. In all its guises, humour and laughter is necessary. It is freeing, it is self-connection, it is a get-out-of-jail-free day pass.

Rolling Forward with Humour

Humour has given me a break from the heaviness, the anxiety, and the weight of a situation. It is as if, in an instant, nothing else matters. Time is suspended.

Laughing at a situation encodes that situation in memory differently—a tough situation becomes associated with lighter feelings. Humour allows me to cope with stress and lessens the negative impact stress has on my physical and mental health. Those high-stress situations affect my morale and my self-talk. They increase my despair, affect my mental health, and can lead to depression.

Humour is a medicine that I've learned can counteract that downward spiral.

Humour also leads to hope, as it offers a release in which I can view situations in different ways. When I can laugh at myself or my situation, I can eliminate related shame. When I see myself through a less serious lens, I can appreciate the quirks of being human.

SEVENTEEN
ALL MY PEEPS

For the longest time, I felt lonely in my grief and my recovery. I was in my head a lot and felt so tired all the time. I also felt like I'd become a burden on others. I couldn't be spontaneous any longer because I needed to plan everything in advance and research accessibility. This meant we couldn't do the things we used to.

I've always had a good base of really good friends. Only a few dropped me after my accident. One group in particular, I call them the Fantastic Six, would regularly check in with me.

Three times per year, we used to go up to my parents' cottage for a weekend. And we'd travel the same road on which I had my accident. Now, not only was the house no longer accessible for me, but the hilly terrain made it difficult for me to be independent—which I hated. So, naturally, these weekend getaways with the Fantastic Six stopped happening.

My friends were undeterred. They invited me to join them in Vegas, or to spend a week somewhere warm and south. I wanted to go but I felt I couldn't. I was stuck in my thoughts that I wasn't good enough anymore. I felt it would be easier for them if they

113

didn't have to worry or plan for me anymore, so I disconnected. Even when we did simple things together, like go to a restaurant, I felt emotionally disconnected. It was like my life was so different to theirs. That feeling lasted years. Until one of them told me that she'd had enough and that I was enough.

She opened up about her fears of losing me when she was told about the accident. She told me she felt I had tuned out. She confided that she didn't want to lose me when I was still here. And then she said I needed to figure it out and come back to them.

So I did. We found an adapted house we could rent on weekends. And we went there twice a year so as to avoid a winter trip—which was a triggering experience for me.

It was hard at first because the girls could stay up later than me. They could drink more than me. They could go in the spa. They could eat anything they wanted.

I felt stuck in that house, but I told myself: at least I was with them. When I faced a new struggle—like the time I needed help in the bathroom—I took thirty minutes before I found the strength to call for help. And they responded in a loving way and helped me clean myself up. No judgment. Just love. And that reminded me of why I had chosen them as my friends in the first place.

I had to learn to adapt and get out of my own way.

Connecting authentically with people, with vulnerability, and sharing my story, my struggles, and my triumphs is not weak, not a pity party, and not attention seeking. And it is not giving up. Let me repeat (for myself): It is not weak and it is not attention seeking.

It is networking. It is healthy networking. It is necessary, healthy networking.

I resisted for the longest time. After all, I knew it all—what could they offer I didn't already know? I also knew that joining groups of people with spinal cord injuries or other wheelchair users would mean that I had accepted *I was one of them*. I didn't want to be one of them. I still held myself as separate: I was a single mom and I told myself these groups targeted many issues, but not parenting. Or some groups were oriented toward athletes in wheelchairs, which I obviously wasn't. There was always something that prevented me from joining.

I was the world's best nonjoiner. At first I resisted accepting a new part of my identity (a mom on wheels, a person with spinal cord injury). I felt I was out of place, the only one fighting for her parenting rights, the only one with a parenting scenario like mine.

A colleague of mine who also works in the field of parenting with disabilities (physical and neurological) suggested I create an Instagram account and follow a few other moms who are also on wheels. As I liked their posts, and commented from time to time, some of these moms started following me as well. I realized I'd started building a community of people with similar attributes. And being part of this online community of moms on wheels helped me understand what I could do with Thomas because I saw what other moms were doing with their kids.

The more I connected with them, however briefly, the more empowered I felt. The more I felt my perspective, my viewpoint, my struggles, and my triumphs were not only seen, but understood. And, most importantly, shared and validated. All of a sudden, I belonged to a group of fierce women who accepted me as one of their own. The more of them I got to know, the more connections I made, the more I began to understand my own legitimacy.

I began to feel like I could be, or maybe I always was, a fierce warrior—not only for me but for them and for others whose voices were not heard. I felt uplifted, growing up and up, where the more women/moms on wheels I saw, the more empowered I felt as I recognized their strengths and their beauty as my own. The more I wanted to get involved and fight for our common human rights, the more empowered I felt, the more I wanted to connect. And the cycle continues.

Connecting with others that may have found themselves in similar predicaments helps us change and grow.

It took me ten years to want to connect with other moms on wheels as a mom on wheels. And now, because I have accepted who I am (a woman with a disability who is a mom) I am truly able to connect and to feel an emotional connection.

I've come a long way from the place where I struggled and felt disconnected from everything and everyone—a place that left me purposeless, directionless, and filled with despair. I didn't know to which group I belonged. My able-bodied friends? My new disable-bodied ones? I felt resentful and, because I was filled with anger, any help that was offered to me felt like a knife in my gut. I wanted to show thanks, but I hated my neediness so much that any offer of help left a bitter taste.

And, in hindsight, that was okay. I needed to go through that. I needed to be honest with my feelings. From that honesty came a way to move forward. When we are our most authentic, we make way for massive progress. When we are our most authentic, we can truly connect.

Rolling Forward to Connect

Human beings are social beings. We thrive in communities. Somewhere inside the memories of our memories are the villages of mothers and children stringing beads, sewing clothes, harvesting berries—insulating each other from peril, sheltering each other from rain, caring for one another and one another's children... leaving no one behind.

Connection includes planning. To look for the best interest for all. For travelling, my plans included inviting along my niece or sister or sister-in-law as a mutually beneficial experience. When we travelled, there would be an extra person or people to help and, as a result, we could all enjoy our connection, and I could learn to accept the help that comes with and through connections, and understand that I was reciprocating in the cocreation of learning and enjoyment for others. We were, in essence, gathered for a berry harvest, the stringing of beads, and the joy of sheltering under the canopy of connection.

We are stronger when we are together, enabling us to tolerate higher levels of physical and emotional pain. When we have the support of others, the worst in life is bearable. Through our villages of connection, our tribes, our friendships, our networks, we find the roots of emotional stability for ourselves and our children.

The more I connect, the more I recognize the strengths and beauty of others as my own.

EIGHTEEN
IT TAKES A VILLAGE

Team parenting—or coparenting—is more prevalent than one might think. It isn't only for us moms on wheels who might need a little extra participation from our village.

It's the "it takes a village to raise a child" phrase that describes a fact that has not changed since, well, since we all lived in villages. In our high-speed urban settings, sometimes the village-style coparenting reality only becomes visible when crisis or tragedy strike, or their opposites: joyful celebrations that bring tears to the eyes of nannies, aunts and uncles, grandparents, neighbours, and teachers when your child (and their child through you) is singing on stage or has an amazing pass-the-puck moment in peewee hockey. Other times, through the everyday stuff, we don't necessarily think about the village. Yet it's there.

The secret, in conscious team-parenting or coparenting, is that your child needs to know who makes the decisions and who to turn to when in need. Helpers, coparents, and other members of the team need to come together on this point so that everyone knows how it is going to work. Life is easier when we are clear about our roles, and that means we're better prepared to adjust and adapt when a situation requiring a plan B or C inevitably comes along.

My coparenting relationship with my mom is strong because my mom truly believes I am the mom.

My parents had been part of the village before my accident, but they were thrust into a full-time coparenting role with Thomas in an instant.

While they dealt with being concerned parents to their daughter (me), her brush with death, and the implications of a significantly changed future, they also had to grapple with the instant and dramatic change in their own life circumstances.

As for me? I had never wanted to coparent—it's why I had Thomas on my own. I had wanted no part of shared parenting, or negotiating when I might have him over Christmas or during summer vacations, I wanted no one-week-on, one-week-off scheduling. I was meant to be his only full-time parent. In a cruel twist of fate, my accident stole everything I had wanted and replaced it with everything I hadn't wanted.

But there was another silver lining that I learned to embrace.

I relied on my parents to support me and, finally, as I was raising a toddler, I realized my parent's continuing support would be wonderful for Thomas and me. I could force myself to do it all and get fatigued, which made me cranky and made it harder to manage my emotions—or I could let my child develop a powerful and wonderful relationship with his grandparents, which enriched his life. I also came to realize that I physically needed help to raise Thomas in the early years and that I wouldn't need that help forever. I knew that it was situational, contextual, and it had a shelf-life.

In those early days when I felt I wasn't truly Thomas's mom anymore, that I couldn't take care of him the way I'd planned, I wondered why I even pretended to try. I disengaged from my parenting role. But I kept returning, because I would notice things my parents did that I didn't like or that I would have chosen to do a different way—like tapping his behind, or too much force around his music lessons.

That's when I realized I needed to take over again. And I began to see how Thomas first came to me for advice, for counsel, and for guidance. I saw the emotional connection he had with me. I saw that Thomas understood that it was mother and son that were a team first, and then we had people who helped us. Loving, wonderful people who held us in a bond of unconditional love but, nevertheless, were not the core team. Through Thomas, I saw the way.

As much as my parents were our life-savers, for which I am eternally grateful, Thomas played a role in making them part of the coparenting team. He knew I was the boss, but he also knew his grandparents would be there for him every time he asked. He also knew what Mamie was good at, what Papi felt like doing, and everything else, including the big decisions, came from me.

Thomas saw us as a collective of love, a collection of mentors, each of us resources he could access. My job was to solidify everyone's roles, establish boundaries, and ensure there was excellent communication amongst all three of us, because that is what is done to succeed. And because his coparents were my parents, I needed to make sure my relationship with my parents would not interfere in our coparenting. In other words, no matter if we had a disagreement, it was important for us to be able to coparent. Which meant our coparenting alliance came first, as Thomas was first. Just like my mom always took care of my needs—even if we had an argument. I was her daughter. Thomas was my son.

As women, the gatherers, the beaders, the shelterers of our modern villages, my relationship with my mom came naturally. Even when I required less assistance, as Thomas grew from toddler to boy, the coparenting continued even as the specifics changed. The village was not going to go away. It expanded just as it does when our children grow and more influences flow into our lives—teachers, coaches, cousins, aunts, uncles, friends, friends' parents.

When I made Thomas, I was prepared and even was looking forward to having him get involved with others: special times with grandparents and aunts and uncles. What I wasn't prepared for was for him to establish a true, intense relationship with my mom. With my dad it was different because Thomas didn't have a father. I wasn't a male figure so there was no risk that my dad might take my place. He had all the space he needed or wanted to take. I didn't feel threatened by it.

But my mom was a mom. My mom. And I was Thomas's mom. And so how would her role, her responsibilities, be different than mine? How would he decipher between Mom and Mamie?

My mom also had a tendency to be a mother figure. But I didn't want her to be. I wanted her to be an extension of me, and a grandma. But not a mother to Thomas. Yet, at times, he needed to have that relationship with her. My aunt, my mom's sister, had taken on the role of a grandmother of some sort. At least, that is how Thomas reconciled it.

I'm sure it was hard for my mom, not knowing where her place was. My dad would get Father's Day gifts and I would get Mother's Day gifts from Thomas. And despite everything she could do for us and with us she didn't have a special day to honour her. All those creative gifts Thomas made were for one person on Father's Day and one person on Mother's Day.

Schools have not yet fully adapted to the fact that there are many kinds of families. Parents and coparents day should be celebrated, instead of a singular Mother's or Father's Day.

There are times when I know she must have felt lost and uneasy. Uncomfortable. Not knowing what she should do or not do. There were times when I resented her: for doing all these things I couldn't do with him. For having those special times that were meant to be mine. Driving him to school, for instance, when Thomas would often have lots to say. And coming home from school, when she would know about his day before I did.

In my situation, there would be times when Mom and I would go on errands and I would open up, or she would. We'd discuss stuff. I'd say what was bothering me, or what I wished would have happened and, in the magical world of mothering power, she would adjust and make a change, and I would make a deal to be more tolerant and accepting of what was.

One of these opening-ups led to my mom saying to Thomas: "This is great, what you did in school, but maybe you should tell Mom first?" She learned to redirect him to me. Just like we had done when he was little. Thomas is now well aware of the things he wants to speak about with Mamie, what he needs to tell me first, and what he wants to say to the both of us.

My mom also learned to redirect all professionals working with Thomas toward me. The eye doctor would want to explain something to a parental figure. An occupational therapist and a speech and language therapist were in nonaccessible offices, so Mom accompanied him. She'd combine myriad statements to make the point that I was his mom: "Don't talk to me, I'm just the driver here." Or, "My daughter is the one who will follow up. She's the one paying you. Please speak with her, not with me. I don't know how she wants things to be done and what things can be done." Or, "I don't understand what you would like me to do; this is not my expertise. Here is her number. I can call her now if you would like. Or you can call her later."

The issues were often at home when I felt my space had been invaded. We are all territorial beings, despite the village atmosphere—just ask any two children sharing the back seat of a car. It's no different for us adults. For me, I would "feel" that my mom or dad would simply enter my apartment without permission —and in hindsight, it makes sense because I was their child. They were my parents. And they were helping me.

Sometimes they would come to wash my clothes or do the dishes, but I didn't like that someone was determining when things should be done and what things should be done. Okay, I hated it. But I was conflicted by the gratitude that they were helping me. In return, my mom often felt I was ungrateful when I'd say something less than what she wanted to hear. There was anger and resentment coming from both of us—and why? Because I wanted to wash my son's clothes. It was something I could do as a parent. It was something many parents would love to have someone else do, but in my tiny world—my perceived tiny world— it was something I could do to show him and to show me and to show the world I was Mom.

The thing about anger and resentment is that it can be contagious. Our children are sponges, we know that, but what they absorb from coparenting mishaps is pretty powerful, just as what they learn from coparenting success is amazing too.

I was teaching Thomas to put away his dishes, and my mom would enter and do it automatically for me and for him. This fired up a reaction in me. And so, Thomas learned to react in a similar way. He'd get angry at his Mamie because it was *his* task. He wasn't doing it just this minute but knew he would do it soon. Taking care of the dishwasher was his chore, for which he would be paid, so he resented it when Mamie hijacked his responsibilities. He too learned to tell Mamie: "No, this is for me to do." And sometimes she would get angry and hurt. For a long time she didn't understand because it was something she was doing out of love. I sometimes had to ask her to "drop it" or "put it back where it was" so Thomas or I could do it.

These kinds of issues will arise when we feel undervalued, or our adulthood is being dismissed and we are relegated to being the child. We have a right to feel frustrated when decisions are made about us without our presence. No matter what our role was prior to being a mom on wheels, we can feel that we have lost important social standing. Dealing with losses while coparenting is challenging. At those times, it is hard to navigate the coparenting relationship.

When we coparent with our parents, then we can fall back into our past relationship of child and parent. I know I sometimes react to my mom as if I was a child, and she can return to the mother-daughter dance we had when I was younger. I have caught myself in a childlike power play, realizing that Thomas was watching, then repeating, my behaviour. I have stayed as alert as possible to let Thomas know that my relationship with his Mamie is different than his and mine and his and hers; we all have a separate identity in our relationships. And at the end of it all, I have to remind myself that in any coparenting relationship, there are going to be struggles. It's not just because I am a mom on wheels.

My coparenting relationship with my mom is strong because my mom truly believes I am the mom. She sometimes oversteps, but not on purpose—she is simply operating on her own mom-ness. When I point it out, she works on readjusting, just as we all must in all our authentic relationships.

As the coparenting evolves, the changes will depend on situations and the child's age, or children's ages. Bring the team concept to the child: they are not the furry mascot on the sidelines, they have a vital position on the field.

As our roles matured, I managed to do things like go to birthday parties (when the party was held at a facility that was adapted) with Thomas. Before we left, I'd remind Thomas that we would do things more slowly than he was used to. We'd take our time, find a solution for every problem we'd face, and that before doing something, we would talk about it. This meant that Thomas had to learn to control his four-, five-, and six-year-old impulses. In the evening or when back at home, Thomas would be a little wilder after controlling his behaviour during these outings. I would need to understand that and be more lenient.

As we started doing more of these things together, Mamie's role had to change. She would come with us to the swimming lessons but, instead of being in the dressing room, she'd be a spectator.

As Thomas got older, division of roles became easier. He could decide for himself who should do what with him—so we follow his lead. He determined that certain things he'd do with my aunt, others with my sister, or sister-in-law, or my brother.

As for the day-to-day roles, we also settled into a certain routine. Mom and I and Thomas live under the same roof, but in separate apartments: my mom has specific tasks to make the house run (groceries, cooking, folding clothes, driving Thomas), while I am the one who makes decisions about things like whether he goes to camp or things that affect his future.

A newer dynamic is that if Thomas doesn't like how Mamie

managed something that happened while she was driving him, he will tell me about it and ask me to fix it. He will say to me, "Talk to your mom, I didn't like it when…"

Yes, the path to clear communication is clear communication—and being responsible for your own words.

When Thomas was younger and had more behavioural issues, my parents and I would often disagree around *how* to parent. Even now, my mom and I can sometimes disagree. For example, Greta Thunberg came to Montreal in September 2019 and I felt it was important for Thomas to attend the march. My mom thought there was not a good enough reason to be stuck in a crowd. Except that I wanted to go, and I wanted to take Thomas even if it meant having him miss school. I almost let my mom's position change mine, but I'm sure I would have later resented it. But I was lucky. My friend Marg had heard me and accepted why I thought it was an important way to teach Thomas about climate change. Because I remained firm in my decision (thanks to Marg), my mom changed her mind. She made it clear she was not enthusiastic about it, but came along anyway because she felt it would be safer for Thomas and me to have walkers around us in a crowd (i.e., bodyguards).

We didn't fight this time. But when Thomas was younger, it happened a few times when I resorted to yelling at my parents as they had done something that I had asked them *not* to do. I also had to ask them to leave the apartment a few times. That was weird for me: I yelled as if I was their parent, while still being their child. I sometimes had to defend my point of view or decision, which I resented. For example, my dad wanted Thomas to play piano. But one year, it got too busy, and Thomas made choices about his activities and music didn't make the list. My dad kept talking about his disappointment that Thomas would not play music. For months, our exchange was like a broken record: my dad would say how sad he was Thomas wasn't playing music, I'd repeat that his schedule was too busy. And then I had a revelation: my dad's disappointment was rooted in a historical disappointment from when I was a child. Which meant this wasn't about Thomas at all. I stopped answering.

Rolling Forward in Coparenting

We all need respite at some time. We might hire someone to clean our home or engage a sitter to watch the child or children for a few hours. Grocery delivery can be considered a kind of respite, as it helps save time. Having someone else take care of your grocery shopping isn't so we can sleep in—it's to liberate us so we can spend time at their hockey or soccer games or ballet classes. But often this is hired help that we pay for. The arrangement is transactional and quasicontractual: they do what we say and we pay them.

Coparenting is not hiring help. Coparenting is dedication, a massive long-term responsibility, and unconditional love. Coparenting is values-based, not a transactional contract but a sacred one.

It helps us to remember this difference when we are making life-changing decisions after we have experienced a life-changing event.

NINETEEN
TOUJOURS PRÊT

Robert Baden-Powell, the founder of the Boy Scouts, coined their motto: "Be prepared." At the time, Baden-Powell was asked what it was Scouts should be prepared for.

"Why, for any old thing," Baden-Powell replied.

Later, he wrote that to be prepared meant to always be in a state of readiness. He believed that Boy Scouts were to be ready, in mind and body, to become leaders and meet challenges with a strong heart. Over one hundred years later, it's still the Boy Scouts' motto.

Translations of this motto echo throughout the world: *Toujours Prêt*, in French; and the Spanish, *Siempre Listo;* and *Sii Preparato* in Italian. And, let's face it, no matter where we are in the world, it's great advice and applies to the safety-pin-in-pocket strategy, and includes everything in between to the often uncomfortable administrative duties such as preparing a will.

As a teenager, I joined the Air Cadets. I fell in love with it: the discipline it required, the belonging and connection I felt, and how it allowed me to expand myself and learn about things I would not have learned any other way. Thanks to Air Cadets, I learned how much I love teaching—how I love finding new ways to spark students. As I gained experience as a survival instructor, our motto, "Expect the unexpected—be prepared for anything," rapidly became mine.

As a cadet, the motto meant being observant, planning for anything that could come our way. It meant getting the gear, knowing where to find information and resources. In one of our survival bush camps with an Army Cadet squadron, all the senior NCOs (noncommissioned officers) were woken in the middle of the night and ordered to pack up our gear in five minutes—we didn't know why, where we were going, or what we would need. We headed out on a nighttime bush walk. At each checkpoint, I would reorganize one element of my pack. At regular intervals I'd look: up at the sky, at the trees, at the terrain. At one point we crossed a road, and I'd paid attention to that, too. About three hours into the walk, our officers asked us where we thought we were. I said: "We have been walking for about three hours, circling back close to main camp. We're close to a town with a population of 60,000, according to the Welcome sign we could see from the road we crossed awhile back."

I didn't really know where we were, but I shared what I did know from my observations. And it was enough to impress my fellow NCOs and officers, and to find my way back if I needed to.

We may not always know where we are going or what will happen, but we can surely pay attention to what is happening along the way, as that might be useful to us at some point.

Twenty years after my Cadet experience, I was in a car accident and I didn't die. As a single parent, I knew I had insurance through work, and I'd checked all the important boxes on the banking and insurance forms—or so I thought. Until I needed them. I saw my work insurance would not have paid out much if I had died. And on the bank's insurance forms, I'd ticked all the boxes except for the one I needed: disability. I would not be receiving any payments to help cover my mortgage.

Thank god my mom and dad were able to pay my mortgage and utilities and to access my bank accounts to pay for things Thomas needed—which they did while I was in hospital and rehab. When I had travelled to Australia in my mid-twenties, I had put my dad on file in my bank accounts as an additional decision maker in all my banking affairs. When the accident happened, that is how my parents were able to continue to pay my bills for me.

In my will, I had previously written that if my parents were alive, they were the ones who would take care of my son, even in the case that I was still alive yet unable to care for him. The accident didn't make me incapable, just unavailable for the first few months as I was in rehab. My checking all the boxes meant that my parents had the legal authority to act on my behalf. If I hadn't done that, child services (child welfare) would or could have been involved.

Living with a spinal cord injury, I certainly learned that life is uncertain and uncontrollable. My survival training in Air Cadets and the "always be prepared" motto stuck with me and reminds me, even now, that anything can happen at any time. And either we learn to think through all the things that can or might go wrong—or we adopt a mindset that says, "when something happens, I will deal with it the best I can."

My sister has four children. Her youngest, Ben, is the funniest kid I have ever met. Bennie and I have a magical bond—it's been there since he was a baby. I was already in a wheelchair when he was born, and often he and I—in highchair and wheelchair—were left together because a certain place wasn't accessible for either of us to join the others. Many times, Ben and I each found ourselves sitting and staring at the other. I learned how to entertain him and we interacted at times and in ways that were unique to us.

Ben and I stayed back while everyone skied. It was easier this way, as my mom and sister already had four young kids to manage. Ben and I spent the day alternating between baking and playing games, with me always having another activity prepared to keep his attention on the here and now and not on "Where is Mommy? I want Mommy!" Preparing these activities was preparing for the unexpected because I was ready to redirect his attention when needed. It saved our day.

Rolling Forward and Travelling Prepared

Six months after my accident, when I attended that first conference in Halifax, we made a list of everything I'd need for my physical care and we found an organization in the city that offered support for people with spinal cord injury. That way, if I needed help, we had the number. We thought we had prepared as much as possible.

The first day, I realized I had a UTI. I hadn't brought antibiotics with me, so my mom and I had to waste a precious six hours waiting in the emergency room so that I could see a doctor and get a prescription for antibiotics. That helped teach me to expect the unexpected, and I now always travel with antibiotics just in case.

Years later, after multiple trips in Hawaii, Australia, Finland, France, and the UK, I learned the value of travelling with a repair kit for my cushion—it got pierced when we were in Hawaii and we were able to immerse it in water, find the hole, and patch it.

As much as I can, I travel with the equipment that makes me comfortable, as it makes the trip more enjoyable and safe. But since equipment needs to be carried, planning a day trip or longer undeniably includes making choices about what I think I might need, versus what I can't go without. Then there's being prepared for when my equipment breaks or is forgotten: my phone can drop on the floor, my chair can get away from me as I transfer from the car. Even in so-called adapted buildings, ramps can be too steep or too narrow and thus be unusable for wheelchairs, toilet stalls may not be wide enough, and, most importantly, ailments associated with my spinal cord injury can occur at any time.

We can travel with tools to temporarily fix our chairs. In my case, my cushion requires air, as do the tires on my wheelchair. I always pack medication and hygiene equipment in multiple luggage cases just in case one suitcase gets lost.

When I know I will be the only adult in the house, or when I travel, I try to think of all the things I may need. Then I make sure these are easily accessible to me, especially if I'm somewhere that does not have all the adaptations my house has. If I'm with Thomas or other children, I make sure I have access to multiple activities to keep them interested, to stave off boredom, and to prevent them from wandering in places I do not have access to. As a last recourse, I make sure I have access to a television or other electronic device that contains several children's apps. Once the accommodation, activities, and potential emergency situations are planned for, I'll talk with the children that are with me. I remind them that there are certain things other adults in their lives can do that I cannot. And I explain that this means there are certain things they cannot do when I am in charge. If they do any of these things and I feel they are at risk, I warn them that we may have to stop any fun things that we had planned to do. Of course, all of this is adapted to the age, maturity level, and trustworthiness of the child(ren). I can do anything I want. I can safely be with children as the only adult—I just need to prepare things differently.

Whether it is the air for tires or the tiny print on travel documents, it all takes on a heightened level of importance for a mom on wheels. On wheels or not, we never know what life will throw at us. For those of us on wheels, we cannot dive quickly (or stand) to catch what is thrown at us. Get real about getting ready for that which you hope will not happen—but could at any moment.

Things just happen, no matter how well I plan for the unexpected. This is just how life is. When I acknowledge and accept that things just happen, I can adopt a mindset that makes me more receptive to solution-finding. Because when shit happens for us moms on wheels, we have no choice but to find a solution—even if said solution is not a great one. We just need to figure things out.

TWENTY
DOG WITH A BONE

In Quebec, the Canadian province in which I live, car accident insurance is legislated to be "no fault." That means regardless of what happened, neither party is considered at fault and every party is entitled to support and rehabilitation for injuries sustained in a car accident. This meant that everything I needed was to be covered by my automobile insurance. Well, in reality, not everything—the role of an insurance company is a rather conflicted one in that they are for-profit organizations that have shareholders. And they don't always part with their money easily.

To receive help from the insurance company, I needed to demonstrate my need, and to demonstrate I needed that help *because* I was in a car accident. The first big hurdle I had with my insurance was about my house.

Those initial days were tough. In our house, the bedrooms and main bathroom were upstairs. So I slept in the space between the dining room and living room, and my parents and Thomas slept upstairs. As a two-year-old, when he had nightmares, my mom would carry him down the stairs so I could be the one to comfort him. Once he'd settled down, she would then carry him back upstairs so he could fall back asleep.

Nothing was adapted for me to be able to change his diapers, bathe him, or cook for us. I couldn't even get into my house on my own as the doors were too heavy. I had no privacy—this was a huge burden on me right there on the main floor. There were so many danger zones for Thomas, we had to have someone able-bodied near us all the time. I wanted my autonomy and my privacy but felt stuck.

The insurance company told me my little house wouldn't be considered adaptable due to the layout and the fact that the adaptations would cost approximately the value of the house. The advice was that I needed to move somewhere else.

I'm lucky to have a mom who is proactive and who understood what I needed to parent my child. She looked for houses in my neighbourhood that would also allow Dad and her to live there—basically a duplex, two homes in one. One morning she announced that she had found such a place. It was one block south on the same street as my house. A duplex with a big yard.

The insurance company did not want to pay for the adaptations to this new house at first. According to their internal rules, when you buy a house and you already have a spinal cord injury, then you need to ensure the house you buy is already accessible for you. In truth, they were hoping I would choose to live in a condo. I advised them that my living in a condo would take my son and me out of my community and standard of living. I'd chosen my neighbourhood because it was family oriented, had lots of parks and easy access to public transportation. Having a big yard was also a bonus as it meant Thomas could play without me having to get to the park, which would require a lot of arm-muscle energy.

I was like a dog with a bone. I wanted and needed a house with a yard. I needed a house that had space for my parents to be close yet not too close. And I needed the insurance to pay for the adaptations. After a few letters signed by my lawyer, they accepted that the adaptation work could be approved on the new house. Once that was approved, I was told the process of adaptation could take up to five years.

Five years! That is not a typo.

This timeline didn't work for me. I was furious. I could not and would not wait five years to take care of my son, and I couldn't pay two mortgages while they determined what adaptations were required.

So, we fought them again. I was still working my rehab program, reentering the work force, and trying to adjust to my new life and situation. I still had regular urinary tract infections which affected my mental health. All this fighting was wearing me down. I just wanted to put my son to bed while he was still little enough that he could enjoy me reading to him and tucking him in.

I was somewhat aggressive toward the architect (who had been hired by the auto insurance company) as I felt he slowed the process, always reminding me that a project of this magnitude could take up to five years. Every time he spoke about the "usual" deadlines, I'd have a crying fit afterwards. How could I be expected to raise my child in these conditions? How could I mother him on my own if I wasn't given the ability? I could only raise my own son if my environment allowed me to. It was incredibly frustrating and took a lot of my energy over the years.

The adaptations to the duplex were eventually complete. And no, it did not take five years. But eighteen months was like a lifetime to me. Thomas was two when the work started, and there's a big difference between a two-year-old and an almost-four-year-old.

I wish there had been another way. One that respected my rights to parent and raise my family the way I see fit, and that would have respected Thomas's rights to be raised by his mother in the environment that was most conducive for his development.

I was grateful to my parents for their own sacrifices—their moving homes. I was able to put some of the fight behind me, which allowed me to choose another challenge.

While I recognize no one intentionally designs a school to be difficult for a mom on wheels, ultimately, the result for one mom on wheels—me—was as if it had been designed to challenge me. But that's the thing with accommodating and adjusting and incorporating and including all people: institutions and the powers that be must be flexible for those they serve—everyone. Every body belongs. I desperately wanted to be able to wheel to the school and drop off Thomas, but the steep hill was impossible for me to roll up, with a child, a school bag, and a lunchbox. Yes, I could drive up the street and drop him off, but I was not allowed to do that. There was a rule that prohibited drivers from turning onto the street during school hours. Understood. It was a safety precaution for the kids. However, residents and others making deliveries were permitted to make that turn. Couldn't they include me, given my circumstances, into their exceptions list?

Apparently no.

I called the city, the police station, and even the ombudsman, and fought for three years to get permission to access that street with my car. I explained to them how it would be even more dangerous for me to transfer out of my car on the busy street down below as I supervised my son.

I was told that, if they gave me permission, they would need to give permission to all parents. I spoke of reasonable accommodations and they said they didn't see the need, as I could always ask any parent to walk my son up the street—basically just hang out and ask another parent to walk Thomas up the hill to school.

Fighting against stubbornness and idiocy was not working for me. I was angry all the time. Pissed off. On edge. And I needed to let it go. In those three years Thomas had grown and we reorganized how I could drop him off. I was fed up with wasting time and explaining everything again and again to people who just did not want to understand.

If I was speaking to my younger self now, I would tell myself: "Marjorie, do your pros and cons on this one. Drop the whole thing sooner. You can parent him without driving him to school. You don't need to do this to be a good mother. Don't hold on to this battle for three years because, in the big scheme of things, your energy can be used to change something else. Please know you are doing this because you have lost so many parts of your role, but you can hear about his day when he gets home. You can create another way to be an after-school ritual."

But somewhere deep down in my heart and soul was also the fact that I couldn't and didn't want to accept that there were different classes of citizens. In my mind, it was anticonstitutional that I, a single woman in a wheelchair, could not access my son's school in a way that was adapted to my physical condition. I still do not think it is okay.

I began to wonder if all the battles are the same in that they all involve a steep hill.

My mom, Thomas, and I decided to drive up to Quebec City for the weekend. We were going to visit some friends who had moved there, and we planned to spend a full day visiting the old part of the city. Between visiting and eating out, we arrived at our hotel room close to ten at night. Obviously exhausted from all our walking—and rolling—we were given a key and then faced with a long list of physical obstacles. The carpet was too fluffy, making it hard for me to wheel myself in. The door did not open on its own and was incredibly heavy. The bathroom sink had a solid vanity under it, therefore my knees could not fit under, plus it was quite high. The toilet was high as well—above the seat of my wheelchair. The beds were close together and too high so I could not get into bed properly. Thomas and my mom had to struggle to lift me while I tried to maneuver my ass onto the bed. I tried not to show my tears to my son but, that evening, I felt a little broken and unwanted.

The next morning, as we went into the breakfast room, Thomas asked me if he could speak with the manager of the hotel. Baffled that my shy son was asking to speak to a stranger, I asked him why.

He said that what had happened the night before was unfair and he wanted to tell someone about it. My son, the shy child who would rather stay in his corner than talk to someone new, wanted to speak out.

I went to the front desk and asked for the manager. When she came out and asked what I wanted to say, she was stunned when I referred her to the little boy beside me.

He spoke very eloquently that morning, explaining exactly what was not accessible and why advertising it as an accessible hotel was wrong. She could only listen. Whether it changed anything at the hotel, I don't know. But Thomas had spoken up in a way he hadn't before. He made me proud.

That day at the hotel in Quebec City, Thomas advocated for all people with disabilities, including me, as he described to the manager how advertising an accessible room yet not delivering on its promises affects all people. It stops people from doing things on their own, and it jointly affects all those who can do things on their own by not addressing privilege.

Through the years, Thomas has been a witness of the fights I have chosen. And by chosen I mean the ones I've participated in and the ones I've walked away from.

This has allowed him to be aware of social justice. I remember telling him about privilege, and what that meant, when he was just five years old. A certain American president had just been elected. I needed Thomas to understand that we were about something completely different. I needed him to be aware that his fair skin, light hair, blue eyes, and male gender makes his journey through life easier than many others as he's unlikely to have to deal with the burdens of discrimination. I wanted him to know that people perceive him differently because of his physical attributes.

There are battles about language. First person—putting the person before stating a challenge so that they are not defined by that challenge—and terminology: disabled, handicapped, and previously used words that are considered much more derogatory and less progressive than the "H" word. The thing is, just like old Uncle Bernie will always refer to something in culture he learned when he was a boy, some words stick around. It's up to a younger version of our population to role-model what is currently accepted and what is currently wanted.

We can use all kinds of terms depending on the trend of the moment, but it is how we interact with people that makes it respectful of their dignity. It is about how we include the person in the conversation and how we make our common environment accessible for all. Dignity and respect, feeling understood, being validated, not judged, is often what is missing in our world. Yet certain words seem to have an impact more than others.

There are some people with disabilities who want to be referred to as being disabled. Others do not. For me, my disability is part of my identity but it is not the sum total of it. I am more than my disability. Which is why I will speak out when someone refers to me as handicapped.

I have limitations, yes. There are things I can no longer do. Yet, provided with the appropriate supports and the right environment, I am able to do much. My disability is mine, but my handicap is ours and it has been bestowed on me by society because society is not fully accessible. My normalcy and my adaptability are arbitrary. To quote a master's degree student of mine, they are "relative and specific to the limited context in which it occurs."

In my house, I do everything on my own. In other places, not so much. We then need, as a collective, to focus on the functionality of the person rather than just labeling with words that do not represent what the person can do, who they are, nor how they can contribute.

TWENTY-ONE
ADAPT-A-PARENT

I n 2016, four years after my accident, I had the opportunity to speak at the Social Work Department of the University of Sydney. I was asked to deliver a speech with the title *Parenting with a Disability: From the Outside In*. Of course, this referred to the fact that, as a scholar, I had studied parenting with a disability from an *outsider* point of view and that now, as a parent with a physical disability, my perspective had changed. What a great opportunity to reflect on the shift from what I knew *intellectually* to what I had come to know *experientially* since my accident.

As I prepared my talk and reflected on what *parenting with a disability* meant, I realized I needed to change the title. I wanted to talk about *parenting with adaptation* instead, because when we label it as *parenting with adaptation*, we base our intervention on the premise that the person offers *good parenting*. It also helps everyone focus not on the disability but on solutions and ideas to support the already assumed *good parent*.

The term *parenting with adaptation* might help us to focus on how we could all support parents like me in doing and being proactive and successful, preventing us, I thought, from focussing on what I and parents like me couldn't do.

Parenting with adaptations could really be a label for every parent, as every parent needs support, respite, advice, counsel, and all kinds of tools and equipment. Some adaptations are common (baby gates and playpens), while others are less so (an adapted crib).

That is what I wanted to convey in that speech: that parenting is the same for everyone, even if parenting by moms on wheels like me may look a bit different.

Of all the creatives and innovators in the world—the sculptors, architects, painters, musicians, and poets—the most creative and innovative of all is the parent.

As parents, we have to find a way to deal with all kinds of challenges because our children depend on us. We have no choice but to be resourceful, think fast, slow things down, and magically make something out of nothing. We invent things—some bordering on the ridiculous, definitely a one-time-fix-never-to-be-repeated, some on the edge of genius, absolutely marketable make-a-million-dollars-from-this idea.

It is what we do. It is not always about finding the best solution, but finding a solution that is good enough.

A solution-finding mindset helped me resolve situations like how to take a shower in a home that is not adapted, or how to turn over in bed when there are no rails—like in a hotel. Even how to purchase and collect Thomas's school books without having to carry the books. And the big one—the one all moms deal with: how to deal with our children's behaviours.

When I was first back home and needed to bathe Thomas, without support, I was presented with the perfect problem-solving, solution-finding challenge.

As I was getting him undressed, he escaped and began running around the house—naked. It was a game to him. I tried to exert my parental authority. Thomas smiled and laughed in the face of my limited success, jumping on his bed, running to the kitchen and hiding under the table—the one place he had already figured out he's safely out of my reach. There he was, in a little ball, taunting me. There was nothing I could do, physically. I couldn't reach him to grab him and pull him out. And he knew it.

I summoned creativity, dismissing the idea of a reward, like coaxing an animal out of a hiding spot with a tidbit of food, knowing that would send us down a road I didn't want to travel. So how else could I coax him out? Aha! I would convince him something else was more fun and that I was having more fun than he was. I grabbed the bubble maker, dipped the plastic stick with the circle on the end into the soapy mixture, and proceeded to blow bubbles as I turned away from the table.

"This is so much fun," I said to no one in particular. "I love bath time because I can make bubbles, and pop them. Wow, I can catch them in my hands."

The more I played, ignoring the naked child under the table, the more intrigued he became. The closer he got to the edge of the table, the further I went. I took my excitement into the bathroom, blowing and popping, and having my own little party. The curious Thomas, enchanted by the bubble game—and wanting in on it— forgot how funny it was to hide under the kitchen table. It wasn't long before he'd climbed into the bath on his own and, at that point, I handed him the bubbles paraphernalia so he could blow his own.

When we create solutions that do not require a physical struggle, or bribing, or exasperation, we grow. We grow in our own estimation and we grow before our child's eyes. They file away the solution-making mom and take the idea with them. This is priceless. Creative solutions take some thinking outside the box, but almost always reduce the stress without causing additional fallout. Many of the things we come up with end up being used again—not just as coping strategies, but—as in the bubbles—as a preventative strategy.

The six months I was in hospital and rehab, and Thomas was being raised by my parents, I was searching for the connection between what was and what was to be. I was a proud single-sole-parent, a full-time worker who also taught two courses, managing while being on call and finding time to be sociable with my friends. It was the whole super-mom enchilada. In the hours after my gruelling physical therapy, my body resting but my mind a bee-hive of activity: what was to be? could I figure it all out? I'd land on a solution to one thing and two more problems would pop into my awareness. Some days I wasn't sure my creative well ran deep enough.

I needed to find creative solutions for situations that got me right in the heart. Like Thomas repeatedly calling my mom "Maman" when I was right there. She'd correct him, and I'd shrivel inside. Yes, she was being his everything, his stability and his support, but *I* was his maman, and she was Mamie. My dad was Papi. They were more than names, and more than roles to me: rather, Mamie and Papi were words that allowed me to be Maman.

Every time Thomas chose to tell or ask my parents something first instead of me, I couldn't help but feel heartache. *Why I had survived the car accident if I couldn't be acknowledged as Mom?* I'd find myself wondering. I couldn't help it. And up would burble feelings of all-consuming sadness, anger—although no one was to blame—and frustration. Sometimes I'd responded by being mean, cutting off my mom, preventing her from answering, being blunt, and reminding everyone that *I* was the mom.

We three adults decided we needed a solution, a way to handle this together so we could all be at peace. We came up with a plan that would make it arduous for Thomas to get anything when he asked Mamie for something when Maman was around, hoping it would help him learn to come to me.

For example, if Thomas asked Mamie for an apple, Mamie would say something like: "Hmmm, Thomas wants an apple. I would love to give him one, but I think there is someone in the house right now who can give him permission to eat the apple. Who can it be? Oh yeah! Maman can!" My mom would then turn back to Thomas and say, "Thomas, Maman is in the room so Mamie will ask her if I can give you an apple." To me she'd say, "Maman, Thomas has asked me for an apple. What do you think? Should I give him an apple? Do I have your permission?"

And I'd respond. "That's interesting that Thomas asked you for an apple, Mamie, as I am right here and he could have asked me directly. But okay, I will answer you. I think Thomas can have an apple as this is good for him and supper is still far away."

My mom would then turn to Thomas and relay my answer. In full. Of course, throughout this whole charade, Thomas would be present—basically doing the child's version of tapping his foot—impatiently waiting for an answer.

It took less than two weeks to flip the switch. Two weeks for my heart to be restored and my parents to feel more at peace.

When we get creative with those who support us, coparent, team-parent, or are temporary helpers, we can empower our children and return the household to a balanced peace.

I had a team of professionals helping to come up with solutions to problems that were mostly environmental and organizational. We managed to find ways for me to change diapers (yeah and yuck). I got to learn how to safely cook so I could make food for Thomas. We explored technology options that could help me push his stroller on my own.

Each creative solution-finding exercise began with the team asking me to define the specific actions I valued as a mother and that were part of my definition of motherhood. From there, we developed a plan to make it happen. They would work with me to readjust either my expectations, or identify how I could gain the physical strength or balance needed through physio, or assess the environmental adjustments that were required. No one ever said to me, "Nope, you can't do that," until we discussed it and tried it.

I sometimes had to modify my thinking. For example, pushing Thomas in his stroller was important to me at first. But as he got bigger and heavier, my choices shifted. The reality of my shoulder strength meant I could either push Thomas in his stroller or go to the park with him or attend his weekend activities. But not all three. Even wheeling myself to the park with him became something that I could do with a little extra help of a battery that I could add to my manual wheelchair. It gave me that extra push. So those solutions came about and were modified as my needs and his needs and my expectations changed. My values stayed the same, but the definition or weight of particular actions got modified as we went along.

Watching us stay focussed and find solutions when things get rough has made Thomas aware that he too can work to find solutions when he encounters a situation he doesn't like. For example, on days when I needed to stay in bed for longer periods of time, Thomas learned he could bring his toys on to my bed. Having him and a jumble of toys including Mr. Potato Head, colouring books and pens, his tea and cookies set, and even his tiny tent with me on my bed actually provided respite for me despite not having much room or peace and quiet.

At just four years old, Thomas asked what he could do to adapt my environment. I answered, wistfully, that perhaps he could build something so that my brain could talk to my legs and vice-versa.

After a significant thinking pause, he said: "We are going to take two pieces of wood that we are going to glue together and that we are going to paint. We then will make a hole and put some wires. We will call the surgeon who repaired your back and we will ask him to open your back again so we can put my machine in. But before we put the machine in, we need to make sure the paint has dried. This is really important. Then, we will do some exercises and sports for your legs, to build your muscles up. That's it!"

He even thought of a solution so that my friend Claude, who is quadriplegic, could cut his own food. Thomas described another piece of wood into which a sharp knife could fit, which would propel the knife and make it cut whatever food was in front of Claude. From a very young age, it was clear that my son had developed the mindset whereby he does not see problems, but sees solutions.

Thomas has many examples of me finding ways to participate in normal activities with some adaptations. He saw me in rehab and has learned that, by adapting things, society becomes more inclusive, and people like me, or my friends, can become more autonomous. A pool could have a special chair to allow people like me to get in. Or, just like Thomas saw, we find ways to adapt to get into the water for his swimming lessons. Yes, I had to transfer onto the floor while everyone was watching me. It was like being a rock star giving a show in Thomas's sold-out tour! He made me feel like a star, by shouting a resounding "Bravo, Maman!" He clearly did not care who was watching. He was just proud of his maman for getting into the pool with him.

Thomas saw the results when we found a special chair that allows me to go into the water. The *Hippocampe*. Depending on the trip, we decide if we bring it or not. And he also saw that sometimes adaptations come from different people. Like on our last trip, one of my cousins, who happens to be an ocean lifeguard, offered to take me in the sea if I wanted to. Four strong men carried me in my chair, over those small pebbles, as close as they could to the water. Then two of them carried me to the water, guarded by my cousin. Everybody watched as we got creative and found a solution.

When we reflect on what parenting with adaptations means to us, as individuals, in our own homes and lives with our own children, in our own family units, we can truly begin to understand the value of creativity, and the role it plays in our lives. Those who came before us have innovated, those who come later—including our children—will innovate. We are the current inventors, solution finders, and modellers of prototypes, all in one person. We are the catalysts for tomorrow's game changers. As mothers, we always will be.

TWENTY-TWO
MIMOSAS WITH FRAGULI

I can face anything head on. I can grunt my way out of a well if I put my mind to it. I can fight my way through rehab to go back to my son. I can do all of that because I learned to savour each moment that life is giving me.

Learned helplessness is a concept I explored in university as I was studying to become a psychologist. It's the process someone can go through that can lead to giving up. I was intrigued with the concept at the time.

After my accident, learned helplessness left a bad taste in my mouth. A bitter taste, the metallic taste of deception and frustration. I had faced and fought against the thoughts I knew would lead to *learned helplessness*. It had become an almost daily fight.

I had to *wait* so often for someone else to do things I could no longer do on my own. I had to accept that whatever I asked to be done would be done differently than how I would have done it. And... I needed to witness it. Sometimes I just wanted to give up because it felt impossible to live with so much frustration all the time.

So many times in rehab, I'd have to wait for one or another of my therapists. I'd feel stuck in the loneliness of this new life—away from my son, from my friends, from my colleagues... every day doing so many foreign things.

Yet, instead of wallowing in the dark thoughts that would creep in every morning and every night, I would find a small hole to park my chair and I'd watch.

I would observe and breathe. I began to focus on what I wanted to see, which was all the beautiful things that were around. I didn't want to see the ugly—I had an overload of that. So I paid attention: to the daughter who helped her mom, to the physio who gently supported her client's legs while asking him to do his transfer as she taught him. I would see the rays of sunshine piercing the windows. I'd hear birds chirping in the trees.

These were my moments of peace, when everything would slow down. The little shift of my mind's eye helped me create my little place in heaven.

Until my physio would signal me that it was time. Time to grunt and lift weights. Time to hurt and sweat. And because I had just spent time exploring the beauty and the good, I would realize it was my good fortune to have the ability to work out. I'd marvel at all the internal sensations, the burning of each muscle—the back muscle or the tiny pectorals that attach under my armpits—and be amazed that I never noticed them work before.

Still, sometimes I did just give up. And breathed, and played *Angry Birds*—to get my mind off the frustration as I learned to wait. I learned to wait until others got it right or until I felt better about having them do things for me.

And I learned that getting things right was not the most important thing. Instead, I learned that doing, trying, learning, being kind to one another, and accepting support from others was all wrapped in love. That was the lesson.

I learned to find ways to feel zen, by meditating and being

mindful of what was beautiful around me. I learned how powerful being in the here and now was. And I learned that everything else could wait.

To avoid the feeling of helplessness that would bring me down, I had to learn to….

…let go of my anger and frustration.

It was cold and dark outside as the Montreal winter weather had crept in, silent and menacing. I was standing in a tiny room in an old hospital, staring at my cousin Sylvia in disbelief.

She had received devastating news: first, she had inflammatory breast cancer. And second, she had just six weeks to live.

I stood there, frozen, unable to comprehend how this could happen to someone like her… positive, energetic, at least until recently. A loving mother who would jump into puddles with her kids, not caring if they all came home soaking wet with water in their boots!

She was my best friend.

The person I spoke to the most.

The one who knew me inside out. And I knew her.

She could cry and scream and it would be a reasonable response. Instead, she established a game plan. She told her oncology team that she needed eight more weeks, not six. Her son's birthday was in six weeks and she had to be there. She would do anything they'd asked, as long as she could be strong enough to be home for Christmas.

Her doctors came back with a plan. They also said it would be brutal. And they weren't lying.

Chemotherapy delivers sucker punches, hitting right where it hurts. Over and over and over again.

But on Christmas Day, Sylvia was home with her children, opening the few gifts she had time and energy to wrap. The next day, she was back for another round of chemo.

She kept her eyes on the prize: more time with her son and daughter.

Then Sylvia asked the doctors for another six weeks—she could not miss the birth of her first nephew. When he was born, she asked for another six... to make it to her daughter's sixth birthday!

Trading in chemo treatments for time and memories, ingesting poison—the price of living just a little longer.

In increments of six weeks, Sylvia made it until just after my son Thomas was born. Four. Years. Later.

Her last milestone.

And when I faced death in that terrible car crash, fourteen months later, Sylvia was there with me. When I wanted to give up and die, she didn't let me. All those years I stood beside her, she had shown me how to live. Her lessons became the blueprints to my own recovery.

As humans, we are wired to fight. And my cousin undeniably showed me how to do just that. Yet her real power, the one that got us both through, was something much more magical.

Sylvia knew how to savour the moments she had, making each new milestone a celebration.

No matter how long—or short—my life is, no matter the struggles I face, I can choose to savour each moment. It's a choice that nourishes hope that other beautiful moments will come my way.

That is what my cousin taught me.

From feeling the sun on my face to holding my son in my arms, I choose to savour every moment. With Sylvia in my heart.

Savouring each moment is not so much an action or a task on a to-do list as it is a stop-between-the-moments and a pause-between-the-breaths kind of thing. It is the sigh that comes from mixing the senses so that we are tasting the meadows and wildflowers, and hearing the softness of velvet against our cheek, touching the pungency of a slightly underripe plum, drinking the colours of a project well completed, and seeing the music as the masterpiece that it is.

Nothing is all negative. In the dark of the night we get to see stars. On the hottest day there is usually some shade. In the wail of our child's tantrum, there is that precious baby of yours, and on your scarred and rough hands—from rolling forward—there is mighty strength.

Throughout my recovery and rehabilitation, I have worked to be cognizant of the little things that are the biggest things in life. I have gotten used to being aware in the way of noting the moments that fill my life, and pausing when certain ones arrive, or shortly after. So small, but powerful, are these moments to be savoured. When it comes down to it, it is the seemingly simple things that catch my breath and capture my heart.

Wrestling and belly-laughing with my son, watching movies with my nieces and nephews, taking a shower and washing my hair —on my own—seeing good friends adapt to my condition, being on my own for a bit, family vacations, writing, enjoying a glass of pink champagne, or a mimosa with Fraguli on the bottom, a special dinner, a brunch, a day outdoors at a campground, meeting new friends who are heart-centred.

These things, and many more, are written in permanent marker on my heart and, in the pauses between the chatter, I let that warm wave called savouring fill my body.

TWENTY-THREE
FORGIVING DAD AND SAYING GOODBYE

My dad always wanted the best for me—and expected nothing less from me.

He wanted me to be a musician. So I learned to play piano. And because I had some talent, and because I would never do anything to disappoint my dad, I practiced relentlessly, every single day. With him by my side.

He would make me run my fingers from one end of the piano to the other, over and over again.

I would learn new pieces and practice those.

I practiced and practiced, with him telling me where I made a mistake and where I hesitated, making me repeat sequences until my fingers could play them without me having to think about it.

Our hard work paid off when I was ranked fourth in the Province of Quebec. I was eight years old and I had played my favourite piece: "The Mouse in the Attic." I had played as if the little mouse was on the keys herself, running up one end of the piano and back down again.

As I stood up to bow after my performance, I could see my dad in the audience, beaming. I had made him proud.

That feeling drove me to continue working hard to achieve *his goals* for me. Until his goals weren't mine any longer, and I told him I no longer wanted to play.

I will never forget that day or the look of incredible sadness and disappointment on his face. I never wanted to see that look again.

Which is why I continued to work toward making my dad proud, to achieve the things he wanted for me.

But after my accident, this time around, I couldn't. No matter how hard I tried.

The frustrating part is that, this time, he and I had the same goal in mind for me: we both desperately wanted me to walk again.

The car accident had severed my spine and my injuries were permanent. Still, I held onto a shred of hope. I held on to the memories of my bodyweight supported by my legs. I worked out harder than everyone else combined in rehab. I gained a reputation for my grunts, my pouring sweat, my disheveled hair, and my look of exhaustion.

And my dad was there. Every day. Beside me. It was as if we had gone back in time, sitting at the piano, practicing and practicing. This time I was doing repetitions of push-ups and sit-ups the way I used to repeat my scales on my dad's favourite musical instrument.

But no matter how hard I tried, I couldn't make his dream come true... *If only I could walk again,* I thought, *maybe my dad wouldn't look so sad. Maybe he wouldn't look so defeated.*

And so I'd push and lift and sweat some more, hoping for either a miracle or that he'd forgive me for not making his dream—our dream—come true.

And then it hit me.

It was time for me to forgive him.

He was the person I most wanted to make happy in the whole world—when I was eight and when I was an adult. And he was relentlessly pushing me to work harder and harder for something I absolutely could not do.

No matter how much he stayed with me while I worked out in rehab, I was not going to walk again.

I realized that sometimes it's the people who are closest to us that want us to become someone or something we are not.

For my own sanity, I needed to find a way to forgive him. I needed to recognize that my dad was human—imperfect and flawed. Forgiving him meant accepting him as he was, the same way I was asking him to accept me the way I was.

My dad only wanted the best for me, his hopes and dreams born from a sincere, incommensurable, and incomparable love for me.

Understanding his motivations and recognizing his limitations helped me let go of the anger and resentment I felt toward him. It released me and brought me to a place where I could love my dad again.

The tulips in Dad's hospital room were a beautiful sunny yellow, standing tall, and commanding my attention. I saw them before I saw Dad.

My dad was a handsome man. With his charismatic attitude, he was often the centre of attention. He loved to tell stories, make jokes, entertain, play music, and sing in front of others. With a guitar in his hands, he was the first person you'd notice in a room. Just like those tulips.

I came to spend time with him every day as I knew these were his last. And as those tulips faded, day after day, so did my dad's health.

He passed away on April 16, 2018. The petals around his tulips had fallen down, one by one, all that was left was their bent-over stems.

When I faced death on January 5, 2012, it wasn't death that scared me. It was the thought of saying goodbye to my loved ones.

As friends and family spent time with Dad during his last few days, I got to see him in a different way. I got to know him in more personal and intimate matters, as he showed me who was most instrumental in his life, whom he still carried in his heart, what affected him and shaped him the most. At the doorstep of death, there were no filters. Everything was honest.

I could sense how my dad wanted to remind himself of the good times and the sad times. How he wanted to share his story. How he wanted us to witness it all so that his spirit and heart and core would live on. Just like the birth of a child, a good death needs to be celebrated. Not in the same way perhaps, but still. Death needs to be part of a more serene ritual of life. His death and life celebrated together.

As my dad took his last breaths, I saw death as a process that included neurons firing in the brain, a *superpower* that allows us to travel from memory to memory and thought to thought, one leading to another and another, making links between people, places, good times, laughter, and sadness. The fireworks these neurons created were emotions linking time and place and loved ones.

In accompanying him in his death, I saw clearly how we human beings are all travelling on our specific road. Even when we live with others, our road is different than theirs. Our choices make our paths different. When we are together, our paths might be parallel to one another, but never the same; separately, our paths shape us differently. And so, I can be a witness to the death of my dad, it can shape me, change me forever… yet, it is not *my* death. It is his. Only his.

My near-death experience on January 5, 2012, was short-lived as I had that yearning to live. But I saw how it affected me. I was not afraid of dying. Just afraid of dying too soon and not being there long enough for my loved ones.

My brain had also fired up my neurons. How else could I have had experienced what I am convinced I experienced in a matter of seconds? My near-death experience triggered those particular memories and feelings to showcase what was most important to me. With that experience, with those memories, I found peace and strength in fighting back. My brain, my survival instinct, and my drive to live showed me what I could live for.

Watching my father's last moments and having experienced my *last moments* in that car have taught me to make the most loving memories during my lifetime. A task that is only achievable if I learn to stay in the here and now. To enjoy my times with my loved ones, to ensure that I act and give my life meaning. Because when death comes knocking again, I would want all those moments of love to fire up the neurons in my brain, so that I leave with the beautiful, peaceful, happy feeling of having lived a full life.

TWENTY-FOUR
WATCHING HIM WATCHING ME

Resilience is having the confidence that no matter what happens, when things don't go our way, we know we will survive, come out on top, learn, grow, and live our lives with purpose. It is the confidence to know that when we fall we have the inner and outer resources to get back up, and that even if we can't get back up we can always crawl. We can keep moving and doing.

Resilience is also being aware that after something bad happens, we may need a moment to catch our breath. And it is knowing it's both okay and necessary to take that time to recover.

When we take the time to recover, we position ourselves to move on and grow, taking in all the lessons the losses have given us. The experiences gift us newfound wisdom.

Resilience is about facing each loss or change with confidence in our capacity to move through it. It's something we practice every time something does not go as planned.

As we practice resilience, we also practice letting our kids believe they are resilient too. We learn to let them explore their own abilities to bounce forward. Instead of always doing for them, we encourage them, support them. We are their cheerleaders and coaches and guides, but we always let them see how capable and strong they are.

And they learn to exercise their resilience by watching us exercise ours.

My purpose is to provide my son with the tools to face each challenge that comes his way, and to build his capacity to create new tools where one doesn't yet exist.

Thomas, my mom, my friend Marg, and I were going to pick apples on a beautiful September day. To get to the apple orchard, we first had to climb a steep hill. Or, they had to climb. I had to roll.

Marg and my mom each asked if they could push me up. "No, thank you," I said. As I was rolling myself up—and it was hard—they kept asking and I kept saying no. Sometimes I would stop, rest, and then roll again. Again they asked until I stopped and told them, "Rolling is my way of staying active. It is good for me physically and it is good for me mentally as I feel I can still do things on my own. For myself. If you want to help, you can stand behind me in case I roll backwards, at which point you can encourage me and believe that I can do it."

I climbed that hill! I was proud of myself and I said so, as we picked our fresh apples.

Weeks later, Thomas, my mom, and I were in the old port of Montreal, heading to an eco-friendly event. Again, I had to face a steep hill. This time it was Thomas who asked me if he could help push me up the hill.

"Do you remember what I said to Mamie and Marg the other day when we were going to pick apples?"

"Oh yes, Maman! I remember," he said. He then called my mom over to stand behind me as he started screaming in the middle of the street. "Let's go Maman! You can do it! A few more rolls and you will be able to get the golden buzzer for your perseverance and determination!" The "golden buzzer" was a reference taken from the show *America's Got Talent*, which we'd been watching lately.

When Thomas faces a hard task, he knows that with perseverance, and by not giving up, he can do hard things. Just like I did. He comes to ask me not to help him, or do things for him, but to encourage him. He knows he learns and feels best when he does things for himself.

During COVID-19 pandemic restrictions, I reopened an 8000-piece puzzle I had started way back at the age of twenty-four. If ever it was the perfect time to work on such a mammoth puzzle, during a pandemic lockdown was it.

Thomas saw me work at it, never letting go, even when the last 300 pieces were all black. Just black. He saw me keep going even when I realized there were pieces missing from the box and that I would never see the puzzle complete. He heard me say that I could not stop because I'd made myself a promise to finish it—not for anyone but me.

I got stuck. I wondered aloud what I should do. I tried different techniques. And I hit another wall and couldn't place any more pieces. Then I'd change strategy and try something new, sharing each stage I was at with Thomas. And I came back day after day.

It took me about twelve hours to place those final 300 black pieces. Thomas was there when I placed the final piece, and he saw the pleasure and pride on my face.

This is how we can teach our kids about resilience and determination and perseverance and creativity and courage.

Children who become resilient become the changemakers of their generation. With resilience comes compassion, and from that comes service. Healthy-minded, balanced children with authentic role models become successful adults.

Postaccident, many mornings I woke, semi-lucid, hoping that I was still in the car. This was my way of wishing I had died. It was how I felt even if I couldn't express it directly. I felt I was a burden on everyone, a liability to all—especially to my son. I believed he was missing out on the opportunities I could not give him now that a wheelchair complicated things for us. I'd get upset because of his waiting for me all the time.

Every two days, I have what we in my house call my long routine. It takes me about ninety minutes longer than my normal routine. On those days, especially on weekends, I need the whole morning to get ready. After spending a week getting up at 5:30 a.m., I can't bring myself to get up that early on weekends, so I start the routine later, finishing between noon and 1:00 p.m.

Everything needs to be organized around my catheterization schedule (the set times I have scheduled to remind me to empty my bladder). For obvious reasons, this is extremely important when I am going somewhere that does not have an adapted bathroom.

All those needs I didn't have before were now in the way of my parenting and in the way of my son's childhood experiences—not to mention a heavy load for those closest to me. If I were dead, I silently thought, Thomas wouldn't have all these complexities. He could have able-bodied parents who would take better care of him.

I felt I was impeding his growth. That feeling lasted a long time. And then, one day, I realized how much my son needed me.

When Thomas was a small child, he needed to know what was

coming next. Perhaps because of my accident, he had (and still has) this ability to think about a bunch of different ways any situation might go. Sometimes he needed reassurance. Okay, often he needed reassurance.

I realized I was the one who could give him that assurance. I was the one who had the patience and time to teach him to be more mindful, to show him how people can be less reactive, and more resilient. I could model it. I could tell him through my actions and my words a story that would stay in his heart forever.

No matter who loves our children—and the more the better— no one knows our children the way a mother does. They are constantly in our sphere of love, a part of us, from us, and they need us. My son needed and needs me.

Having two able-bodied parents would not mean Thomas would have a better home, or that he would be better supported. It was up to me to provide the best environment he needed in *my* home. In *our* home. And again, with this realization, my incredible love for him fuelled my resolve to keep going despite the despair I sometimes felt. The more I felt reassured by the notion that I *was* the best parent for him, the more I was infused with motivation to do things to keep me safe and healthy. I knew I could do it, because I was doing it, and because I had been doing it since his birth.

I was a rolling example of resilience.

All the kids around me have learned that I can pretty much do anything I want to, with perhaps a few adaptions. My nephew Max and I have adapted our basketball games—sitting on a chair. I swim with everyone, and wear my floaters in case one of them tries to hold on to me. Children have asked to push my chair to help me;

some of the little ones have learned they can sit on my lap when their legs hurt. We have adjusted to table activities instead of playing on the floor. We located the *real* adapted cinemas and love going—it has become our favourite activity. We found new ways to race each other: them running, me rolling after them. They have adapted to our new normal!

They also see things differently. They notice more things than their peers who are not around moms on wheels. When my niece got a doll house with three floors and an elevator for Christmas, she turned around to her mother and said, "There's an elevator for Auntie Marjorie!" When Ben was little (he's the youngest of our family), he would listen intently to my voice when I helped him get out of his highchair. He would wait when I told him to. He knew he needed to listen to my directives to be safe. We could stay together for hours, just the two of us, and there were never any issues. I loved those special moments with Ben—especially when he was the same age as during the months I lost with Thomas.

Those moments show me that both kids and adults can adjust and demonstrate resilience. Since Thomas was two years old, I adapted to my new physical abilities, which allowed me to spend quality time with all, including Ben. At six years old, my nephew feels safe with me. When he wants to take a walk in his neighbourhood just with me, we go. Once, he saw me struggle to get on the sidewalk, and right away he came to offer help. He then walked toward the park and kept announcing big and small obstacles on the sidewalk.

As for their perception of all of this: as long as I laugh with them and tend to their needs, they don't seem to care that I do it while sitting in a chair rather than standing. And when I can't get something for them, say, if it's too high, they have learned to climb onto my lap and reach for it themselves. Teamwork.

Raising healthy, resilient children really comes down to trusting them that they will focus on what really matters, and trusting ourselves to let them work most things out—or be involved in the troubleshooting. This teaches them how they can contribute, making them more accepting, inclusive, and involved citizens.

TWENTY-FIVE
ROLLING FORWARD

When I couldn't find another mom on wheels role model to show me the way, I turned around to see if there might be others following in my wheel tracks, watching me become the person I want to be for my son. You'll notice I said "become" and not "be." Because it is a process. A journey. I'm showing him that I want to become a better person, not that I am a better person.

One evening at supper time, Thomas grabbed his phone and starting surfing social media. (His phone has no SIM card for phone service, but it uses WiFi for the signal.) I immediately reacted, telling him to put the phone aside—which he did.

A few minutes later, he took out his phone again.

"Why is it so important that you absolutely have to check your phone right now, while we're still eating?"

He ignored me and continued to use his nonphone, but he was measuring my anger. As my face became hotter and redder, because he wasn't listening to me, he said, "I wanted you to feel what I feel when you take out your phone and look at it."

"I don't do that! Not when you are with me."

Thomas said nothing. I reiterated that social media and apps and phones and technology were not welcome at the supper table. As we transitioned to dessert, and Thomas brought the dishes to the dishwasher, I suddenly caught myself. I had picked up my phone to check for notifications.

I was mortified. I hadn't noticed this about myself. Thomas had.

As we were eating dessert, I asked him if he had been feeling bad about me picking up my phone at the table for a long time. He confirmed he had.

I apologized and I asked him to tell me next time he feels he doesn't like something I do, so I can fix it sooner or explain it if I can't fix it. We agreed.

Thomas, my mom, and I entered quarantine March 10, 2020—a few days earlier than everyone else in Montreal. I'd heard that some children had been confirmed or suspected of having COVID in Thomas's school. Since both my mom and I were in what they called "vulnerable" groups due to our age or physical condition, I didn't want to take any chances. I was more at risk because I can't cough. My lung capacity is seventy percent as my abs cannot push on my diaphragm.

Thomas agreed to see people only via a screen or far away in a park. He stopped doing any activities with friends, and organized himself to be an online student. A month went by, then another, then it was a year, then we were at eighteen months. Although he was a trooper in disrupting his whole life, we could see that it was making him scared. An already pretty anxious boy, he was now really worried that I could die… again. For him, the whole COVID experience brought back feelings he probably didn't know he had. What would that mean if I died? Who would take care of him? Who would be in his corner? Who would guide him?

COVID also brought some of my own fears back up: fears of dying, of leaving Thomas. It was my posttrauma that I did not want to seep into him, but I wondered if it had since we were both fearing anew the same things.

I noticed Thomas being hard on himself, feeling badly if he did something in a way I didn't want, or if he forgot to finish some schoolwork. Even when I told him it was okay, that he'd soon learn to be more organized, he still judged himself harshly. He didn't realize that the lockdown had stretched thin his tolerance and inner resources.

Then it dawned on me. He was using the same self-talk I had been using when I felt incompetent as a mother or as a person.

COVID laid our nerves bare, rendering them hypersensitive. It was harder for us to control our anger or frustration. A lot of little things triggered reactions that were out of proportion for the event. I knew that we were not going to survive long-term stay-at-home orders if we did not change something. And so, on a walk outside one day (distanced and wearing masks of course), I could see Thomas' stress come out.

"You should relax, Thomas," I said, trying to be helpful.

"Well maybe *you* should learn to relax too and show me how it's done." His hot reply shocked me. At first. Then I realized he was right.

I realized Thomas was reproducing my behaviours, following my lead, and not listening to my advice (do as I say, not as I do!). If I wanted him to grow up with the strategies in his toolbox to make him a more centred and mindful human being, I needed to become a person who is more centred and mindful. I needed to change. I realized that the skills I wanted Thomas to have were the skills I needed to learn myself. Which meant I needed to learn and apply them.

We both needed to learn to centre ourselves. We both needed to find effective strategies for the triggers coming our way. And we both needed to find a way to lower our reactivity levels.

Thomas had been doing yoga at school, but it wasn't part of the online learning experience. He had some coordination issues and couldn't follow online yoga classes—they caused more frustration than anything else because he couldn't understand what movement was expected.

So I told him about meditation and then about mindfulness. We followed meditation classes together. We established an evening routine to include a gratitude journal and an eight-minute meditation. We did this routine together, and we added additional sessions separately. For example, I adapted my own version of a body scan (no body-scan meditation exists for someone who is paraplegic) to awaken me in the morning. He did a recentering meditation at noon or right after his online schooling.

Because I love learning, I studied, read, and trained in mindfulness meditation whereby I focussed on character strengths. For example, I used my curiosity to explore how I relate to my legs now that I don't feel them the same way. My perspective helps me dance with my arms: moving each finger, being present in the movement, in the resistance with the air. And I celebrate! I celebrate my arms and the fact that I can move them.

Incorporating mindfulness and practicing meditation did a few things in my life. First, I was less reactive. I could hear my thoughts and knew how they could trigger a behaviour I would not be proud of. For example, if a bowl was dropped and I saw Thomas hustling, unsure of what to do next and nervous of my reaction, I would hear a stream of thoughts. *Shit, now I need to clean that up. Cleaning something from the ground is hard for me! All the small pieces of glass could puncture one of my tires! I'll have to call my mom to do it for me. I hate asking for help! Asking for help makes me weak and just shows how useless I have become.*

With those thoughts came the feelings of hopelessness and anger and translated to me asking Thomas to "clean it up fast" to relieve my negative thoughts about myself. Because I spoke impatiently, Thomas would assume I was mad, he'd cry and then not be able to pick it up as he was too upset. I'd then hear myself say something like, "Oh come, no reason to cry, it's just a bowl."

It was amazing to me how practicing mindfulness helped me see all of that unfold as it was happening. As I practiced, I got better at refraining from saying certain things, changing my tone of voice, or simply stopping and giving him a hug.

Mindfulness provided me with the ability to change the course of my thoughts as I became aware of them and of their impact. My knowledge of my character strengths led me to knowing I had the personal resources, like self-regulation or perspective, that led me to make more mindful choices.

As I did that, the house became a more tranquil space—the air seemed to be filled with kinder and more compassionate thoughts than it had been.

Thomas adjusted to and started practicing mindfulness and meditation on his own, when he felt he needed it. Thomas learned to manage his anxiety better, was able to interrupt his bouts of anger before they happened, and we both started to take things less personally, which liberated us to have more open conversations.

Parenting is truly about supporting our children to be the best version of themselves. One way of doing it is to become the adult we want our children to be.

When we move on with our lives, there is no place where we suddenly stop moving on. Breakthroughs happen, growth happens, then more shit happens, and the cycle of learning rolls on.

The problems I had to face right after I was given my wheels may have seemed insurmountable at the time, and there was lots of advice offered that things would get easier. And some things did.

Life and parenthood are lived with a moving target—a growing child—and there will always be challenges, whether or not I'm a mom on wheels. Whether it's a car accident or—or something else, there will be other adjustments to make. They may not require masks, but they'll likely still require tissues, and chicken soup, and compassion—especially for the self.

EPILOGUE

T he auto insurance people wanted me to drive again. My rehab team wanted me to drive again. My parents felt it would be better for me because driving again would give me increased autonomy.

I hated all of them for saying that. Until I started having post-traumatic reactions as a passenger. I reacted when my mom turned left on a two-way street. When my dad would drive too fast… when the wind would move the car… that feeling of *whoosh*… bringing me back into *that* car. I'd see the other cars coming my way, I'd focus on the lights, seeing them as light beams from the truck. I'd relive the intense fear of those seconds before impact. Even as I write this… I am taken back there. In my car. Unable to do anything. Helpless. Unable to move. Paralyzed. By fear. Physically. Emotionally. Cognitively. I know what is coming and… tears roll down my cheeks.

Eighteen months after I fired that first psychologist, I agreed to see another. But only to help me get back behind the wheel of a car.

I chose this psychologist carefully. She was the friend of a friend

—that's how it happens sometimes. She was the only one I would trust. The only one I would let in. So we made a plan.

She helped tremendously. She helped me fight my fear and challenge my thoughts. But everything in our work together was geared toward me driving again. And we were successful: I began to drive again and I drive to this day.

When I first went back to work, I was burying my feelings of what being paraplegic meant, what sharing custody of my son meant, what incontinence was doing to my soul. They were soul-crushing. I didn't deal with those feelings, and then when I lost my ability to work too, it was like a tsunami. All those feelings sending me tumbling, swirling, unable to breathe. It was the second event I could not control. It was terrifying.

I met another psychologist, and two weeks after I began seeing her I went on sick leave. I started seeing her, dealing with all those feelings, too late to save my job. But I continue seeing her to this day.

Those feelings were deeply rooted in those irrational thoughts of mine. Those preconceptions of what needing help meant. With this new psychologist's help I identified those thoughts, challenged them, learned to choose which thoughts I could absorb and act on and which to turn away from.

I know those thoughts can be triggered easily, and at any point. I know how to recognize them.

But now I also know something even more powerful: positive psychology and character strengths. This is the approach that should be used—in my personal and professional opinion—in rehab centres everywhere. Because knowing we all have twenty-four character strengths that we can tap into at any point, for every situation, gives us back our power. It certainly gave mine back. And that is what I needed: to regain my own power.

An example I often give is this. When I saw the car, I knew that was it for me. I was meant to die. I first thought I could not do anything to change that. With the knowledge of positive psychology and character strengths, I was able to see that I used love (my top, most often-used strength) to summon my will to survive. I used prudence (a middle strength of mine) as to not aggravate my injuries when I told myself to stop moving and wait for first responders to do their thing. And I used spirituality (my least-used strength) to ask to have my arms back and to know I was not alone. It gave me the perspective that I had something to do with surviving and having use of my arms. I had always had some control over how I react, over my thoughts, and my behaviour. I could have made it worse but I didn't. I helped myself. Even in the most terrifying and helpless moment of my life: I had control over me. And that made me powerful. And useful.

In any given moment, I can choose to use my strength of creativity to think of a new solution, my strength of love of learning to learn a new way of doing things. At any given time, I can leverage my strength of teamwork to raise my son with my parents, my strength of kindness to feel connected to others. Every single chapter of this book is about one or more of these strengths, how these character strengths were useful to me, how they made me better and stronger.

This is what is needed in the rehab world. I am telling you.

ACKNOWLEDGMENTS

To feel compelled to write is one thing, to do it another, and to share is something completely different in and of itself. I would never have thought my stories could be shared if I had not been seen for who I am despite and with my new acquired disability. To all the professionals from Sacré Coeur Hospital, l'Institut de Réadaptation Gingras-Lindsay de Montréal, la Clinique Parents Plus, and le Centre de Réadaptation Lucie Bruneau who supported me, taught me, took care of me (and continue to do so): you saw me as a person with dignity who deserved your time, your expertise, your interest, and investment. You saw me as more than just a body, broken and whole. And you recognized my strengths and believed in me when I certainly did not think I could.

Sharing my most intimate and vulnerable moments would also not have happened without the encouragements, cheers, and faith shown by my friends, many of whom are healthcare professionals themselves. Numerous times they have shared about how my stories impacted them as my friends but also as workers. To Melinda, the "head cheerleader" of my cheer squad. To Laura, my "parents with intellectual disabilities" partner, the greatest rights advocate and my friend, for reading the second major revision and providing invaluable comments and suggestions. To Marg, for making such a significant difference in my life and in so many others. No matter the role you take on—nursing, spiritual leader, social worker, coparent, cheerleader, or advocate—the one that has impacted me the most is your role as my super-friend. Thank you for reading two major versions of this manuscript and providing me with strong and thought-provoking remarks and suggestions. This manuscript would not be what it is without your input and your faith in me. To Vanessa, for offering a true and real perspective of the value of this manuscript, for giving me suggestions to ensure every writing piece has a clear purpose.

To Gwynnyth, an incredibly talented, valued, internationally praised researcher and advocate for parents with disabilities, for providing many invaluable seminal pieces of research in the field of parents with intellectual disabilities and for normalizing and bringing forward the key concept of community and support (without shame nor guilt). In Capetown, in a bar with our esteemed friends and colleagues in this world of parenting and disability, you made a statement that reinforced and reassured me: I could become a single parent by choice, because a child needs at least *one* adult that believes in them to grow up strong and resilient. I knew my baby to come would have me, and my community—so I knew he would grow up fairing more than okay. And in Halifax, years later, when you met him, you reassured me again that parenting with disabilities—all kinds of disabilities, including spinal cord injuries—is possible, and that we should teach our kids lessons that will make them more creative, justice driven, and kind. And that is something we should all strive for. So when you *asked* if you could read my manuscript, it certainly was a great honour for me. You allowed me to believe I *can* do anything I set my mind to! And for that, I will be eternally grateful!

In the northern hemisphere's summer of 2020, I was interviewed by Caroline, a high school friend, for Mothersphere, a social media group for mothers to connect and be inspired. She and Tanya thought mothers around the globe would benefit from hearing my story. By asking me, you opened up windows and doors to what is now my new life, I will forever be grateful to you! Sharing my story with Caroline and Tanya led me to Speaker Slam and to sharing stories of my life with Universal Messages that impact. To Dan and Rina, cofounders of Speaker Slam and my friends, you have created a powerful platform and have embraced me in your community. Being part of it all has shaped my writing to be purposeful. Many of the stories I shared in my speeches are represented in this book as they have truly been pivotal in my life. Thank you for guiding me through to the me I am now!

The more I shared, the more I gained in confidence, a confidence that led me to reaching out to Fatima Doman, the author of *Authentic Resilience*, a book that gave me tools and strategies to reframe how I had previously seen my predicaments. Thank you Fatima for your kind words and for being so certain that my story needed to be told and shared.

As I reframed and was trying to make sense of where I was and what my life had been since my accident, the science behind positive psychology and character strengths (VIA Institute) gave me a lens with which I can make sense of my disability in a different, more empowering, hopeful way. Ryan and Ruth were my teachers and guides in this process as they gave me the vocabulary and tools to use and recognize how my strengths of perspective, bravery, appreciation, and gratitude have made a difference in my life. I will forever be appreciative, grateful, and blessed for their friendship! As for Stephanie and Lydia, cofounders of the Hope Warriors Podcast, they have reminded me that I could see events as happening to me, or focus on how I was still able to pull in my own internal resources. Through conversations with them and Ruth and Ryan, I realized love had saved my life, prudence had protected me from further injury, spirituality had kept me sane and peaceful even when I thought I could no longer move my arms, and hope had led me to recovery. They helped me see I had everything in me already. Thanks to your influence, I have reconnected to a spiritual life that helps me stay grounded even in a place with regular earthquakes.

When everything shakes, including our own confidence in ourselves, it is great to have friends that know and are convinced of our worth (and who constantly remind us). Emmanuelle is this friend for me. From high school, when we maybe spoke ten words to each other, to a phone call received by my mom a few weeks after my accident, to a friendship that has now lasted more than ten years! You have been my rock and my safety net on numerous occasions and made sure that the lioness in me still had that ability to roar loud and strong about the unfairness and discrimination my new disability brought with it. You have given me peace of mind more than once by making it known you were standing beside me. You introduced me to Joe, a lawyer who works in the literary world, and this is how I met Boni and John at Ingenium Books!

I also had the chance to meet amazing people in my life, some with whom I connected right away. Ian and Maria are those great giants I feel blessed to have met and worked with. To Ian Tyson, the ace in my deck of cards. Working with you on several of my speeches was an honour and a blessing! To Maria Sirois, it was such a privilege to learn from you about the whole process of storytelling and about positive psychology and resilience. Your wisdom has transformed my life in more ways than one, and you have touched my heart forever.

To my publisher Boni: working with you has led to some pretty challenging times when I definitely had to learn to relinquish control and trust the process you led me on, yet I feel tremendously privileged to have had the opportunity to work with you. Your ability to synthesize and take the wider view and decipher what is relevant and useful in the whole story is incredible and I thank you for the journey. To Marie, for being there, behind the curtains. I know how hard you have worked to make sure my story was framed so that everyone can relate.

To all the moms I worked with, especially the moms of the *Parenting Group*, who have always shown me how it is done. To Julie (not her real name), the first mom I met, and to Star (also not her real name), the single mom who inspired me the most in my whole career.

To Evelina, my "parents with disabilities" partner, working with you provides me with great joy and a strength beyond what I could have imagined! You introduced me to a few moms on wheels, which led to meeting up with more moms on wheels—and that simple act has given me a sense of belonging that I had lost in that car. Knowing and seeing all those beautiful mamas is making me stronger than I thought I ever would as a mom on wheels. You gifted me with one of the most precious gifts: the feeling of worth, identity, and pride. So to all of you, moms on wheels and future moms on wheels and parents with disabilities, thank you for your friendship and for putting your stories out there to inspire all of us: to @soleinedemetre_leoniepoudrier, @morenikego, @daniizzi, @happy_para_mum, @adaptiveparentproject, @marcogpasqua, @christacouture, @blindmotherhood, @disabledmums, @eliza-hull, and all the ones I have not met yet.

To paralympian, gold-medalist and Senator Chantal Petitclerc for your support in amplifying the voices of parents with disabilities and for sharing positive parenting from a wheelchair! Your encouragement and validation have meant a lot. I never thought I could compare to what you have done, until I realized that it is not a competition—but rather it is about us supporting the endeavours of others. This is how we change the world. Thank you for your support and teaching me this beautiful lesson. And thank you for inspiring me to be better, do better, and to rejoice for what I have.

To my newest most brilliant friend Ingrid Palmer @focusonability-life, you have shown me how to roll forward with pride as a woman and mother with a disability, and for that I will eternally be grateful to you. Your friendship gives me energy and joy.

To my closest friends, whose lives changed with mine, who adapted as I did, who accommodate as my disability is now part of their world too. You have made me feel less alone and have given me strength when I didn't even have enough for myself. You have been there for Thomas when I couldn't and have embraced my parents as your own. There are no words to tell you how blessed we are to have you in our lives. To Sophie, Anne-Marie, Stephanie, Paula, Kelley, Kelly, and Jan I love you. And to Alexandre, Peter, Richard, and Pierre, all the men in (y)our lives, I thank you for the impact you have on my son and I celebrate the men that you are. To Melissa, Isabelle, Amanda, Rosa, Carol, and Lisa for your continued friendship. You were front and centre when my life changed course and you adjusted as I did, never letting me behind.

When I was transported to the spinal cord injury-specialized centre in Montreal, my loved ones were all going back to their homes after a week of joy and love spent altogether. Yet they all rallied to my hospital gurney as soon as they heard. They took care of my son when I couldn't. They made sure I knew I was not alone. They held each other so that together we would not fall. My brother Fabrice made sure to be a dad figure with his stupid dad jokes and play fights. Always there to make sure we had space to connect and have fun—together. *Never* leaving me behind. Always ready to hold me up, pick me up, refill my rum and coke, paddle our kayak, and always letting me know I matter and I am loved. To my uncle Christian who lets me know he cares, not in words, but in so many other ways. He and my aunt have supported my cousin the way my parents have supported me. The parents behind the mothers. Becoming more than grandparents but without ever aspiring to become parents to their grandchildren, yet providing love, care, safety, and a place to belong. Making my cousin and me the best moms we could be. Tata, Tonton, all my life you have been like second parents to me—caring for me as one of your own. I am so grateful to have you in my life and I love you more than words can say.

To my dad and his petit père, who are, for Thomas and me, the men who have had the biggest impact in our lives. My dad will always be my hero: a kind man with strong values, who loved his children more than anything in the world and who would have done anything to protect them and ensure their happiness. His infinite love he shared with his children and grandchildren, passed on from his petit père and grandmother to him, to us.

The idea to pursue single-motherhood by choice was a conscious choice on my part. A decision that took several months and years of reflection. It was about identifying my values and beliefs and going for my dreams, enabling my hopes for a future I longed for. I could not have even imagined single motherhood if it hadn't been for all the wonderful mamas in my life who have inspired me. My mom, tata Badette, my cousin Sylvia, my sister, and sister-in-law are the ladies who I look up to the most. If I made the choice of becoming a soloparent, it is because I had seen how my world is managed by the most beautiful and resilient mothers there are. You have shown me that the love that comes from being a mum and grandma can make us most vulnerable yet give us this out-of-this-world strength: this love allows us to go beyond who we are as a person and woman. This tender and fierce motherly love allows us to find out who we are, makes us learn new abilities, dictates the tough choices we need to make, and teaches us to breathe through our noses when the situation requires it. I am truly blessed to have such beautiful role models.

To the mother behind the mother: my mom. The one person

who has been my legs and my arms more times than I can count. You have given me life, loved me, and raised me. You have let me go so I could travel on my own journey, and when I needed you most, you were there to ensure I could parent and raise my own child. Thank you for being in Thomas's parenting circle. For loving me and loving him the way that you do.

And to the only one who made me a mom in the first place: Thomas. I understand that at twelve years old, we don't want our moms to openly say they love us, but writing a book is a big deal, so you will have to accept that I am telling everyone how much you mean to me and how incredibly blessed I feel to have you in my life. You are the single most important person to me. You were a dream I carried in my heart for so long and you shaped me into the woman I am now: the strong, resilient, proud mom on wheels.

ABOUT THE AUTHOR

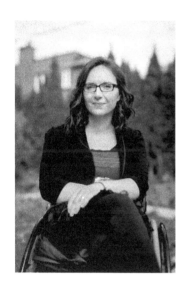 Marjorie Aunos, PhD, is the Speaker Slam North America Speaker of the Year (2021), and an author, internationally renowned researcher, clinical psychologist, and adjunct professor at Brock University and Université du Québec à Trois-Rivières. She is the chair of the Parenting and Parents with Intellectual and Developmental Disabilities Special Interest Group (SIRG) of The International Association for the Scientific Study of Intellectual and Developmental Disabilities. She developed the first program offering support for families headed by parents with intellectual disabilities in Quebec, Canada. In 2012, while at the peak of her career and mother to a sixteen-month-old boy, she sustained a spinal cord injury in a car accident.

Marjorie believes that focussing on our strengths of character can lead to living a fulfilling life. She is the coauthor of *Comprehensive Competence-Based Parenting Assessment for Parents with Learning Difficulties and Their Children*. Marjorie is bilingual in English and French.

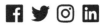

BOOK CLUB BONUS

We recommend taking *Mom on Wheels* to your book club. Get your reader's guide for book club discussion questions here: https://ingeniumbooks.com/mow-bookclub.

BIBLIOGRAPHY

Angelou, Maya. *Letter to My Daughter*. New York: Random House Publishing Group, 2009.

Aunos, M., Hodes, M., Llewellyn, G., Spencer, M., Pacheco, L., Jareslàtt, G., Tarleton, B., Springer, L., & Höglund, B. (2020). "Chapter 14: The Choice of Becoming a Parent." In *Choice, Preference, and Disability: An International Perspective*. Springer Publishing. R. J. Stancliffe, M. L. Wehmeyer, K. A. Shogren, & B. H. Abery (Eds)

Brown, Brené. *The Gifts of Imperfection: 10th Anniversary Edition*. New York: Random House, 2020.

Chödrön, Pema. *When Things Fall Apart: Heart Advice for Difficult Times*. Boulder, Colorado: Shambhala Publications, Inc., 2016.

Devine, Meghan. *It's OK That You're NOT OK: Meeting Grief and Loss in a Culture That Doesn't Understand*. Boulder, Colorado: Sounds True, 2017.

Doman, Fatima. *Authentic Resilience: Bringing Your Strengths to Life!* USA: Authentic Strengths Advantage, LLC, 2020.

Esfahani Smith, Emily. *The Power of Meaning: Finding Fulfill-*

ment in a World Obsessed with Happiness. Penguin Random House Canada, 2017.

Feldman, M. & Aunos, M. (2010). "Comprehensive Competence-Based Parenting Assessment for Parents with Learning difficulties and Their Children." NADD Press. (Out of print.)

Frankl, Victor E. *Man's Search for Meaning*. Boston, Massachusetts: Beacon Press, 2006.

Hahn, L. (2020). "The Well-Being of Youth Brought up by Parents with Disability: A Longitudinal Population-Based Study." Thesis. Edmonton (Alberta, Canada), University of Alberta, Doctor of Philosophy in rehabilitation Science.

Hone, Lucy. *Resilient Grieving: Finding Strength and Embracing Life After A Loss That Changes Everything*. New York: The Experiment, LLC, 2017.

Kingsley, Emily. *Welcome to Holland*. 1987.

Kushner, Harold. *When Bad Things Happen To Good People*. New York: Anchor Books, 2004.

Lopez, Shane. *Making Hope Happen: Create the Future You Want For Yourself and Others*. New York: Atria Paperback, 2013.

Mercerat, Coralie (2021). «Analyse de l'adéquation entre les besoins des parents vivant avec des limitations physiques et les services en périnatalité et petite enfance.» Thèse. Montréal (Québec, Canada), Université du Québec à Montréal, Doctorat en Psychologie.

Neff, Kristin. *Fierce Self-Compassion: How Women Can Harness Kindness to Speak Up, Claim Their Power, and Thrive*. New York: Harper Collins Publishers, 2021.

Niemiec, Ryan M. & McGrawth, R. E. *The Power of Character Strengths: Appreciate and Ignite Your Positive Personality*. USA: VIA Institute on Character, 2019.

Pausch, Randy. *The Last Lecture*. New York: Hyperion, 2008.

Pituch, E., Ben Lagha, R., Aunos, M., Cormier, T., Carrier, A., Gagnon, C., Gilbert, V., Dominique, A., Duquette, A., Turcotte, M., Wakil, R.-M., Bottari, C. (Submitted). "What Services?: Perceptions of Key Stakeholders on Early Support Needs for Parents with Neurological Disorders." *Disability & Society*. (ID: CDSO-2022-0112)

Reivich, Karen & Shatté, A. *The Resilience Factor: Seven Keys to Finding Your Inner Strength and Overcoming Life's Hurdles*. Three Rivers Press: Random House, Inc., 2002.

Sandberg, Sheryl & Grant, Adam. *Option B: Facing Adversity, Building Resilience and Finding Joy*. New York: Alfred A Knopf, 2017.

Sirois, Maria. *A Short Course in Happiness After Loss (and Other Dark, Difficult Times)*. Housatonic, Massachusetts: Green Fire Press, 2016.

United Nations' Convention on the Rights of Persons with Disabilities. https://web.archive.org/web/20220520004245/https://www.un.org/development/desa/disabilities/convention-on-the-rights-of-persons-with-disabilities.html (retrieved March 15th 2022).

Wolbring, G. (2008). *The Politics of Ableism*. Development, 51(2), 252-258.

RESOURCES

CHILDREN'S BOOKS:

Mama Zooms by Jane Cowen-Fletcher
Dad Has a Wheelchair by Ken Jasch & Anita DuFalla
Mom Can't See Me by Sally Hobart Alexander
We Move Together by Kelly Fritsch & Anne McGuire
Some Days: A Tale of Love, Ice Cream and Mom's Chronic Illness by
Julie A. Stamm

BOOKS:

We've Got This: Stories by Disabled Parents by Eliza Hull
How to Lose Everything by Christa Couture
Maternity Rolls: Pregnancy, Childbirth and Disability by Heather
Kuttai
*Disability Visibility: First-Person Stories from the Twenty-First
Century* by Alice Wong
A Celebration of Family: Stories of Parents with Disabilities by
Dave Matheis

REPORTS:

Rocking the Cradle: Ensuring the Rights of Parents with Disabilities and their Children. National Council on Disability

MEDIA:

Fathers with Learning Disabilities. Moore Lavan Films. (YouTube)
Being a Parent: Parents with Learning Difficulties. ParentingRC. (YouTube)
We've Got This: Parenting with a Disability. Eliza Hull, ABC National (Podcast)
Insider's Guide to Pregnancy and Paralysis. Dani Izzie, Reeve Summit Webinar (YouTube)
Dani's Twins. Dani Izzie (Documentary Film)
Ouch! BBC (Podcast)
La parentalité après un accident. Accessibilité Média Inc. (YouTube)
The Barriers, Both Physical and Social, I Face as a Parent Living with a Disability. CBC First Person (Online Article)
Des Familles comme les autres. Animé par @guylou avec @evelinapituch. La parentalité après un accident. Accessibilité Media Inc.

BLOGS:

https://blindmotherhood.com
https://blindmomintheburbs.com
https://makingitontheplayground.com

ASSOCIATIONS:

The Association for Successful Parenting (TASP) Twitter: @TASP2009
International Association on the Scientific Study on Intellectual and Developmental Disability (IASSIDD), Special Interest Research Group (SIRG) Twitter: @parentingsirg
IG: @iassiddparentingsirg
Parenting with Intellectual and Developmental Disabilities

SERVICES AND PROGRAMS:

Canada
Surrey Place (Toronto)
Sunnybrook: Adapted Maternity Clinic (Toronto)
Centre for Independent Living in Toronto (CILT): Parenting with a Disability Network (PDN)
Clinique Parents Plus (Québec)
Tetra Society (Chapters Across Canada)
National Federation of the Blind
Spinal Cord Injury BC

United States
The Disabled Parenting Project (Brandeis University, MA)
Help Hope Live
Center for Research on Women with Disabilities (Baylor College of Medicine, Houston, Texas)
Through the Looking Glass (California)

Europe
Together Parenting Project (Surrey, UK)
Working Together with Parents Network (Bristol, UK)

ASVZ (Netherlands)

Australia
Healthy Start and the Parenting Research Centre. Twitter
@parentingr

FACEBOOK GROUPS:

Irresponsible Father's Guide to Parenting
Disabled Mums (Australia)
Diversability Community
CILT Parenting with a Disability Network
Parents with Disabilities
Les mamans d'exceptions
Groupe de discussion – parents en situation de handicap
(QC)
MobileWOMEN
Parent roulant!

CPSIA information can be obtained
at www.ICGtesting.com
Printed in the USA
LVHW051533240622
722062LV00005B/466